SYSTEMS OF THE HUMAN BODY

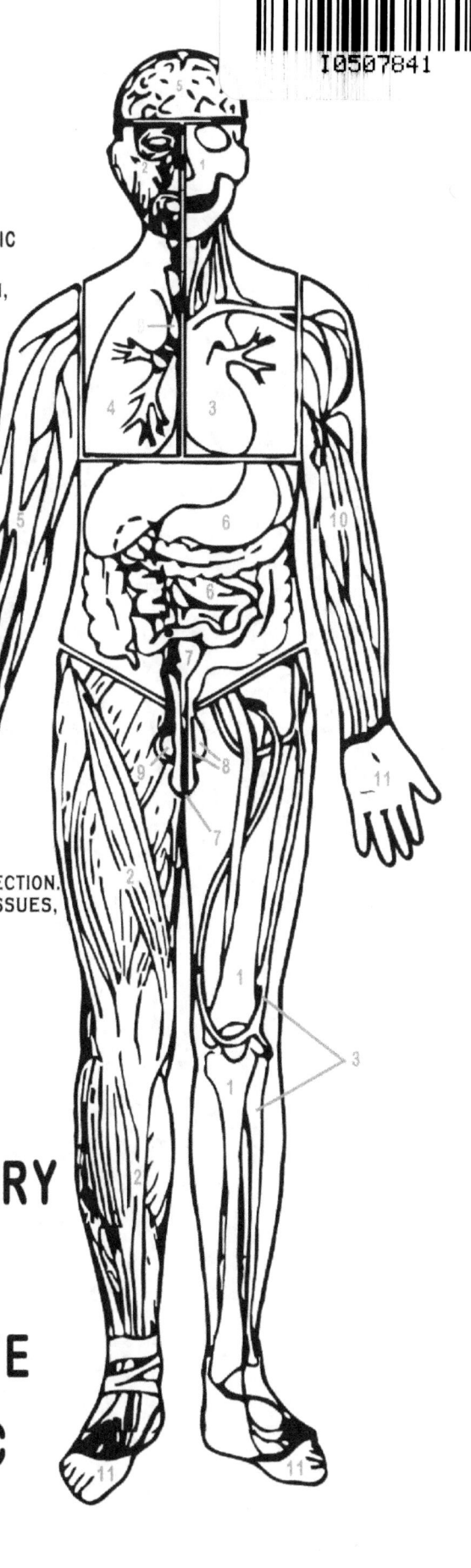

OUR BODIES CONSIST OF A NUMBER OF BIOLOGICAL SYSTEMS THAT CARRY OUT SPECIFIC FUNCTIONS NECESSARY FOR EVERYDAY LIVING.
THE JOB OF THE CIRCULATORY SYSTEM IS TO MOVE BLOOD, NUTRIENTS, OXYGEN, CARBON DIOXIDE, AND HORMONES, AROUND THE BODY.
IT CONSISTS OF THE HEART, BLOOD, BLOOD VESSELS, ARTERIES AND VEINS.

THE DIGESTIVE SYSTEM CONSISTS OF A SERIES OF CONNECTED ORGANS THAT TOGETHER, ALLOW THE BODY TO BREAK DOWN AND ABSORB FOOD, AND REMOVE WASTE. IT INCLUDES THE MOUTH, ESOPHAGUS, STOMACH, SMALL INTESTINE, LARGE INTESTINE, RECTUM, AND ANUS. THE LIVER AND PANCREAS ALSO PLAY A ROLE IN THE DIGESTIVE SYSTEM BECAUSE THEY PRODUCE DIGESTIVE JUICES.

THE ENDOCRINE SYSTEM CONSISTS OF EIGHT MAJOR GLANDS THAT SECRETE HORMONES INTO THE BLOOD. THESE HORMONES, IN TURN, TRAVEL TO DIFFERENT TISSUES AND REGULATE VARIOUS BODILY FUNCTIONS, SUCH AS METABOLISM, GROWTH AND SEXUAL FUNCTION.

THE IMMUNE SYSTEM IS THE BODY'S DEFENSE AGAINST BACTERIA, VIRUSES AND OTHER PATHOGENS THAT MAY BE HARMFUL. IT INCLUDES LYMPH NODES, THE SPLEEN, BONE MARROW, LYMPHOCYTES (INCLUDING B-CELLS AND T-CELLS), THE THYMUS AND LEUKOCYTES, WHICH ARE WHITE BLOOD CELLS.

THE LYMPHATIC SYSTEM INCLUDES LYMPH NODES, LYMPH DUCTS AND LYMPH VESSELS AND ALSO PLAYS A ROLE IN THE BODY'S DEFENSES.
ITS MAIN JOB IS TO MAKE IS TO MAKE AND MOVE LYMPH,
A CLEAR FLUID THAT CONTAINS WHITE BLOOD CELLS, WHICH HELP THE BODY FIGHT INFECTION. THE LYMPHATIC SYSTEM ALSO REMOVES EXCESS LYMPH FLUID FROM BODILY TISSUES, AND RETURNS IT TO THE BLOOD.

CHOOSE YOUR OWN COLORS
1. SKELETAL   2. MUSCULAR.
3. CIRCULATORY   4. RESPIRATORY
5. NERVOUS   6. DIGESTIVE
7. URINARY   8. REPRODUCTIVE
9. ENDOCRINE   10. LYMPHATIC
11. SKIN

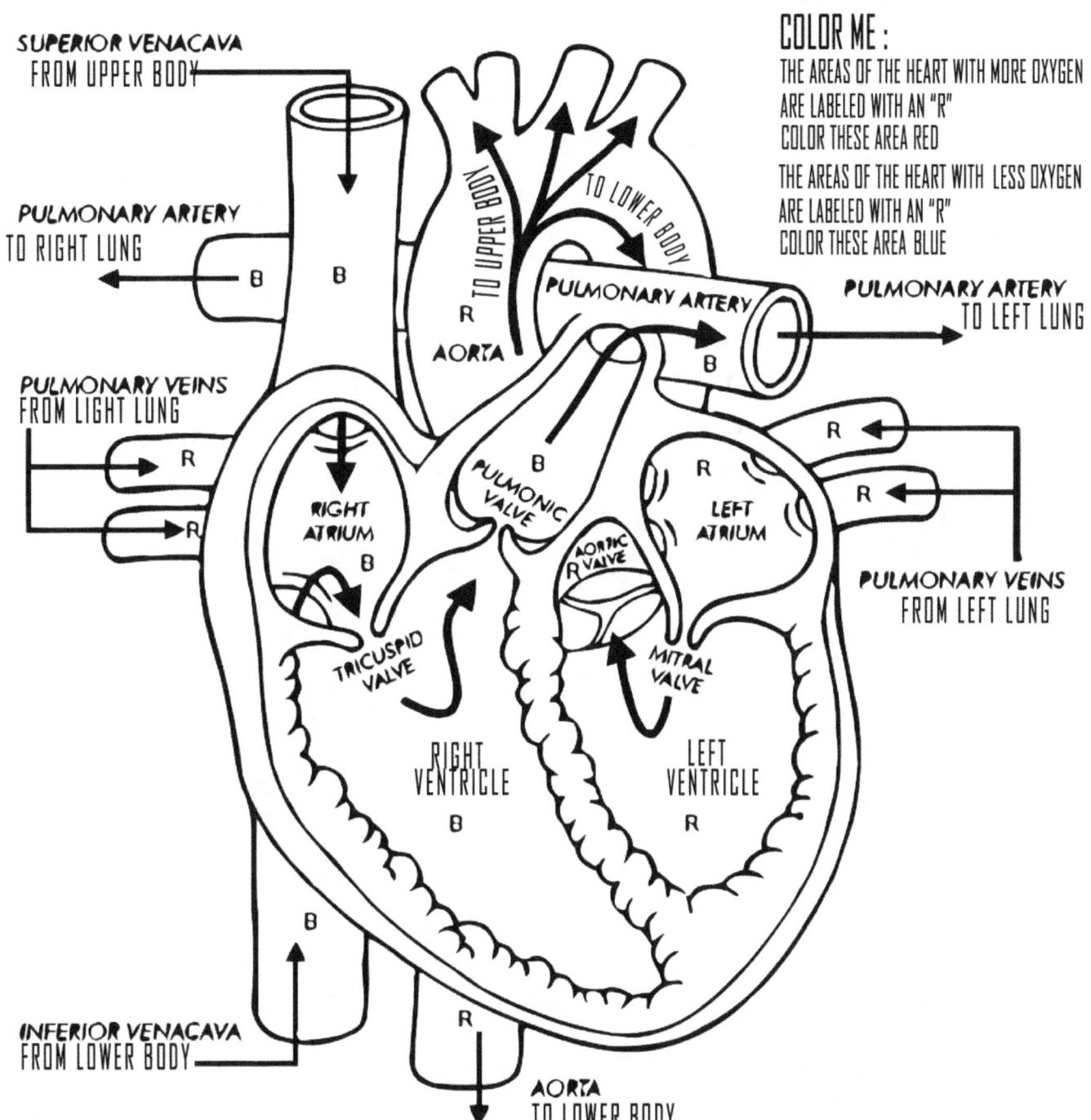

Pulmonary Circulation

IS THE PORTION OF THE CIRCULATORY SYSTEM WHICH CARRIES DEOXYGENATED BLOOD AWAY FROM THE RIGHT VENTRICLE, TO THE LUNGS, AND RETURNS OXYGENATED BLOOD TO THE LEFT ATRIUM AND VENTRICLE OF THE HEART. THE TERM PULMONARY CIRCULATION IS READILY PAIRED AND CONTRASTED WITH THE SYSTEMIC CIRCULATION.
THE VESSELS OF THE PULMONARY CIRCULATION ARE THE PULMONARY ARTERIES AND THE PULMONARY VEINS.

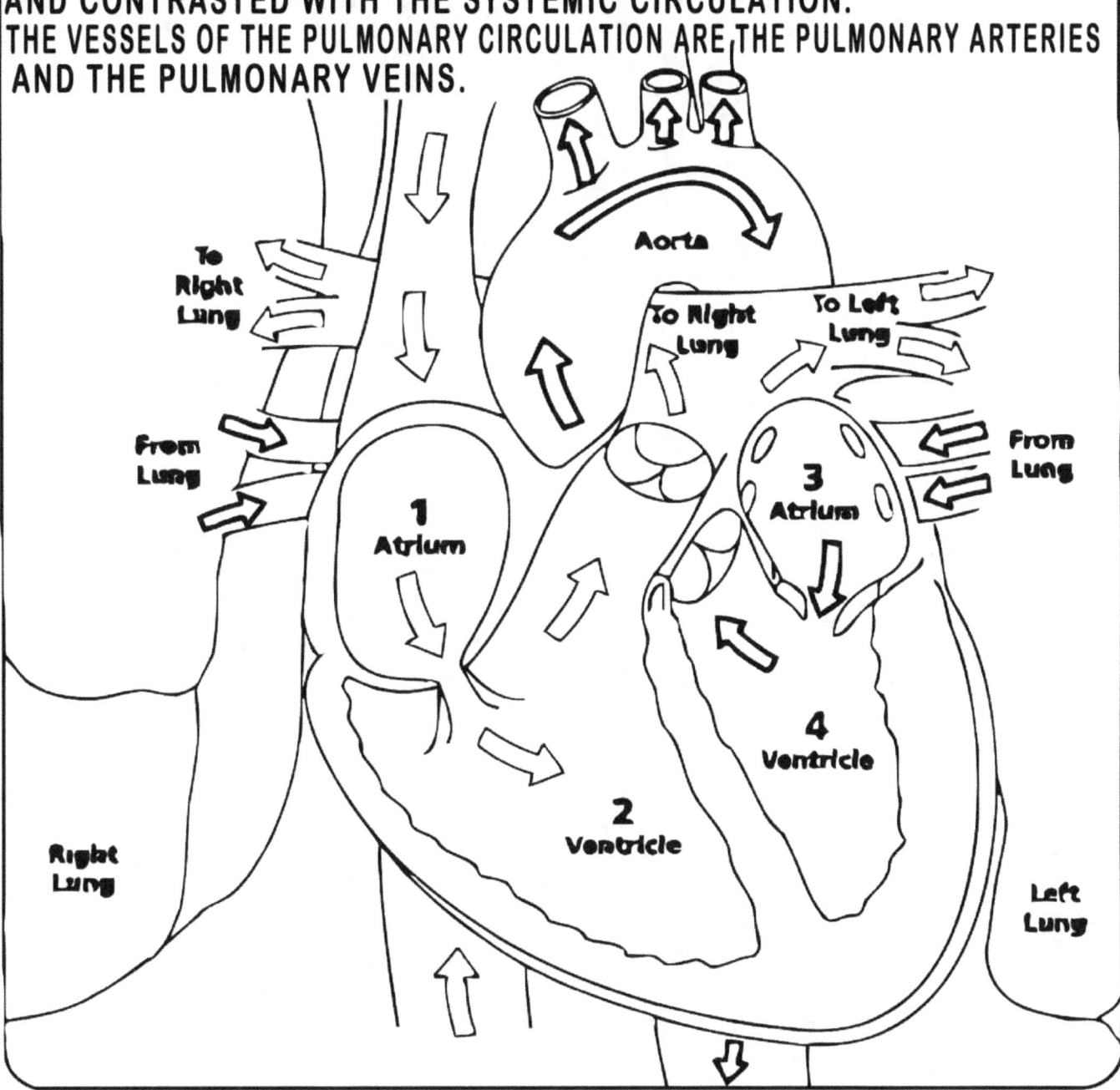

STRUCTURE OF THE NEPHRON

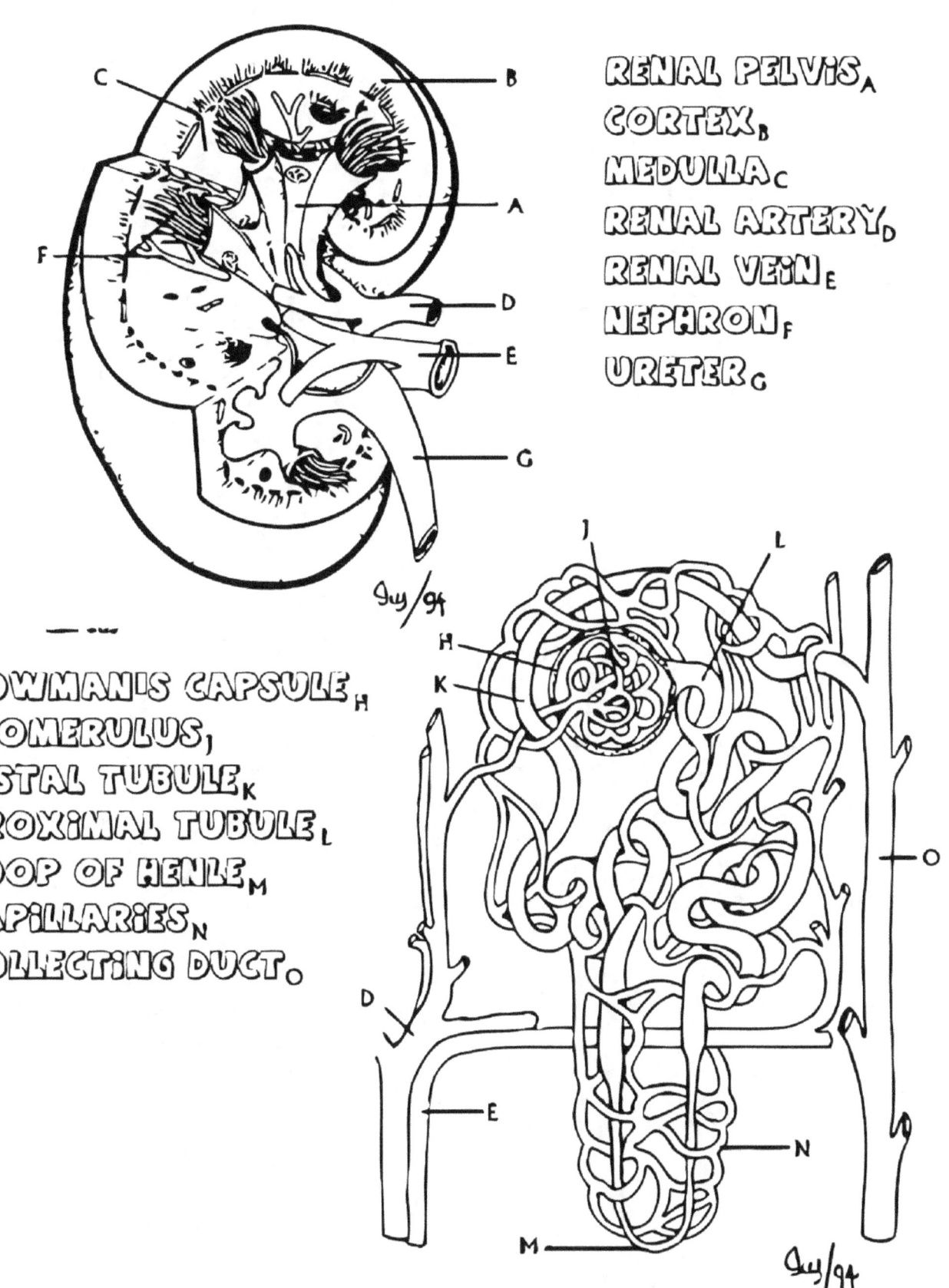

RENAL PELVIS A
CORTEX B
MEDULLA C
RENAL ARTERY D
RENAL VEIN E
NEPHRON F
URETER G

BOWMAN'S CAPSULE H
GLOMERULUS J
DISTAL TUBULE K
PROXIMAL TUBULE L
LOOP OF HENLE M
CAPILLARIES N
COLLECTING DUCT O

SKULL

THE SKULL IS A BONY STRUCTURE THAT FORMS THE HEAD IN VERTEBRATES. IT SUPPORTS THE STRUCTURES OF THE FACE AND PROVIDES A PROTECTIVE CAVITY FOR THE BRAIN. THE SKULL IS COMPOSED OF TWO PARTS: THE CRANIUM AND THE MANDIBLE. IN HUMANS, THESE TWO PARTS ARE THE NEUROCRANIUM AND THE VISCEROCRANIUM OR FACIAL SKELETON THAT INCLUDES THE MANDIBLE AS ITS LARGEST BONE. THE SKULL FORMS THE ANTERIOR MOST PORTION OF THE SKELETON AND IS A PRODUCT OF CEPHALISATION—HOUSING THE BRAIN, AND SEVERAL SENSORY STRUCTURES SUCH AS THE EYES, EARS, NOSE, AND MOUTH. IN HUMANS THESE SENSORY STRUCTURES ARE PART OF THE FACIAL SKELETON.

HYOID BONE

THE HYOID BONE (LINGUAL BONE OR TONGUE-BONE) IS A HORSESHOE-SHAPED BONE SITUATED IN THE ANTERIOR MIDLINE OF THE NECK BETWEEN THE CHIN AND THE THYROID CARTILAGE. AT REST, IT LIES AT THE LEVEL OF THE BASE OF THE MANDIBLE IN THE FRONT AND THE THIRD CERVICAL VERTEBRA (C3) BEHIND

PARIETAL BONE	PINK
FRONTAL BONE	TURQUOISE
LACRIMAL BONE	GRAY
ZYGOMATIC BONE	BROWN
NASAL TURBINATES	RED
TEETH	LIGHT BLUE
NASAL BONE	BLUE
MAXILLARY BONE	LIGHT PURPLE
MANDIBLE	ORANGE
SPHENOID BONE	YELLOW-GREEN
TEMPORAL BONE	GRAY
OCCIPITAL BONE	YELLOW

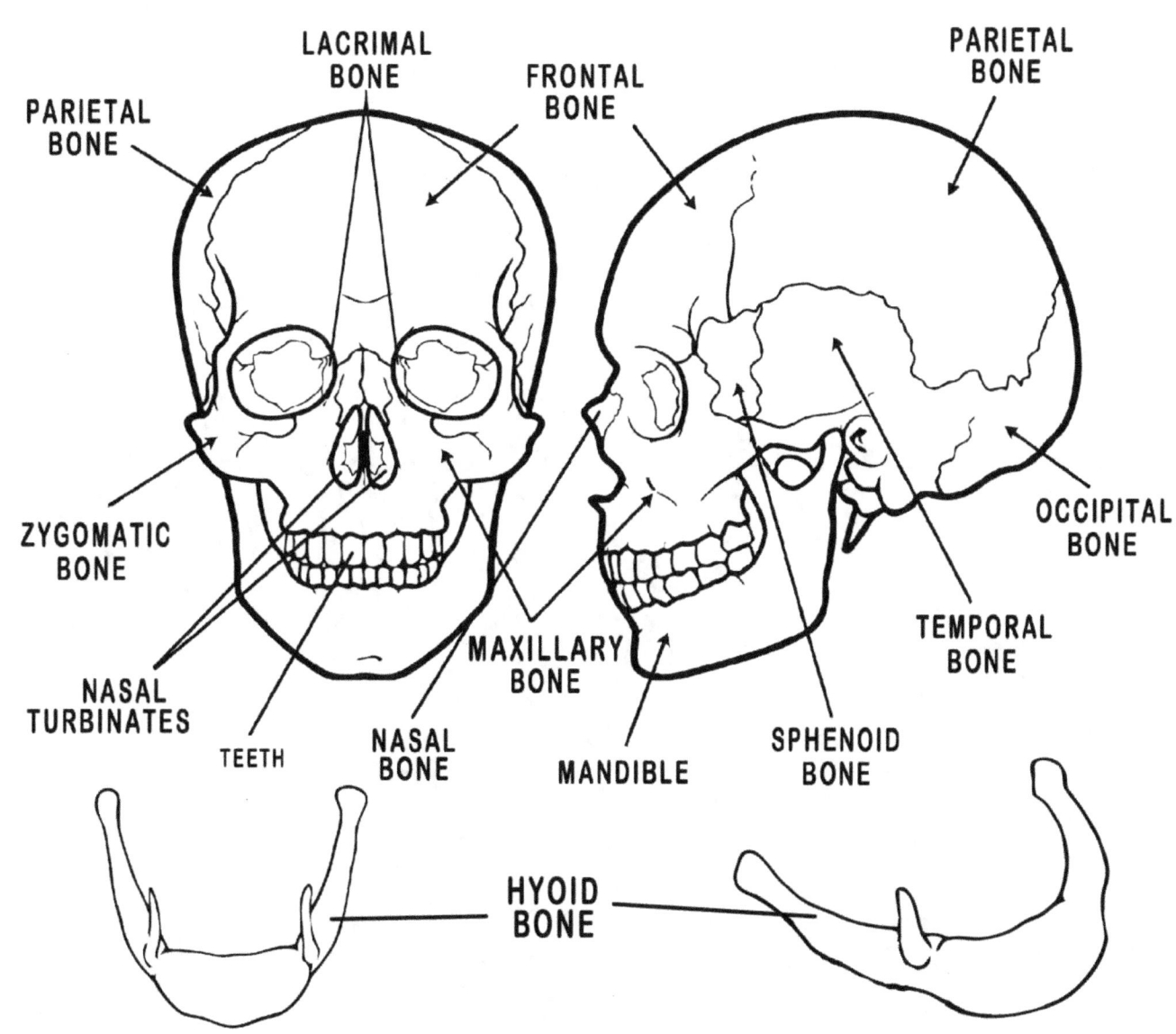

SKELETAL SYSTEM

THE HUMAN SKELETON IS THE INTERNAL FRAMEWORK OF THE HUMAN BODY. IT IS COMPOSED OF AROUND 270 BONES AT BIRTH – THIS TOTAL DECREASES TO AROUND 206 BONES BY ADULTHOOD AFTER SOME BONES GET FUSED TOGETHER. THE BONE MASS IN THE SKELETON REACHES MAXIMUM DENSITY AROUND AGE 21. THE HUMAN SKELETON CAN BE DIVIDED INTO THE AXIAL SKELETON AND THE APPENDICULAR SKELETON. THE AXIAL SKELETON IS FORMED BY THE VERTEBRAL COLUMN, THE RIB CAGE THE SKULL AND OTHER ASSOCIATED BONES. THE APPENDICULAR SKELETON, WHICH IS ATTACHED TO THE AXIAL SKELETON, IS FORMED BY THE SHOULDER GIRDLE, THE PELVIC GIRDLE AND THE BONES OF THE UPPER AND LOWER LIMBS. THE HUMAN SKELETON PERFORMS SIX MAJOR FUNCTIONS; SUPPORT, MOVEMENT, PROTECTION, PRODUCTION OF BLOOD CELLS, STORAGE OF MINERALS, AND ENDOCRINE REGULATION.

THE HUMAN SKELETON IS NOT AS SEXUALLY DIMORPHIC AS THAT OF MANY OTHER PRIMATE SPECIES, BUT SUBTLE DIFFERENCES BETWEEN SEXES IN THE MORPHOLOGY OF THE SKULL, DENTITION, LONG BONES, AND PELVIS EXIST. IN GENERAL, FEMALE SKELETAL ELEMENTS TEND TO BE SMALLER AND LESS ROBUST THAN CORRESPONDING MALE ELEMENTS WITHIN A GIVEN POPULATION. THE HUMAN FEMALE PELVIS IS ALSO DIFFERENT FROM THAT OF MALES IN ORDER TO FACILITATE CHILDBIRTH. UNLIKE MOST PRIMATES, HUMAN MALES DO NOT HAVE PENILE BONES.

SHORT BONES: IS ONE THAT IS CUBE-LIKE IN SHAPE, BEING APPROXIMATELY EQUAL IN LENGTH, WIDTH, AND THICKNESS. THE ONLY SHORT BONES IN THE HUMAN SKELETON ARE IN THE CARPALS OF THE WRISTS AND THE TARSALS OF THE ANKLES. SHORT BONES PROVIDE STABILITY AND SUPPORT AS WELL AS SOME LIMITED MOTION.

LONG BONES: IS ONE THAT IS CYLINDRICAL IN SHAPE, BEING LONGER THAN IT IS WIDE. KEEP IN MIND, HOWEVER, THAT THE TERM DESCRIBES THE SHAPE OF A BONE, NOT ITS SIZE. LONG BONES ARE FOUND IN THE ARMS (HUMERUS, ULNA, RADIUS) AND LEGS (FEMUR, TIBIA, FIBULA), AS WELL AS IN THE FINGERS (METACARPALS, PHALANGES) AND TOES (METATARSALS, PHALANGES). LONG BONES FUNCTION AS LEVERS; THEY MOVE WHEN MUSCLES CONTRACT.

FLAT BONES: IS SOMEWHAT OF A MISNOMER BECAUSE, ALTHOUGH A FLAT BONE IS TYPICALLY THIN, IT IS ALSO OFTEN CURVED. EXAMPLES INCLUDE THE CRANIAL (SKULL) BONES, THE SCAPULAE (SHOULDER BLADES), THE STERNUM (BREASTBONE) AND THE RIBS. FLAT BONES SERVE AS POINTS OF ATTACHMENT FOR MUSCLES AND OFTEN PROTECT INTERNAL ORGANS.

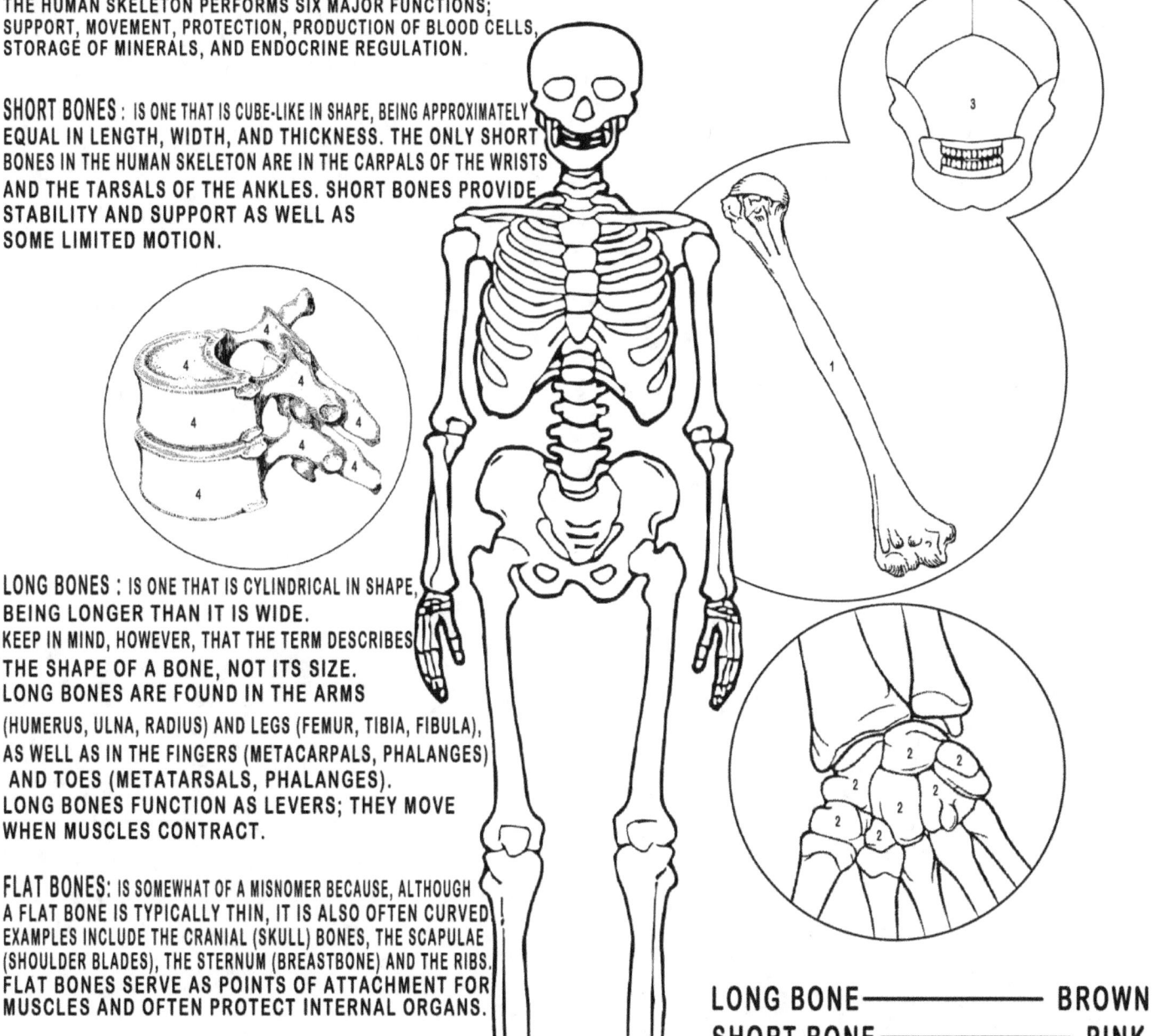

LONG BONE ———————— BROWN
SHORT BONE ———————— PINK
FLAT BONE ———————— BLUE
IRREGULAR BONES ———— YELLOW

VERTEBRAL COLUMN SPINE

ALSO KNOWN AS THE BACKBONE OR SPINE, IS PART OF THE AXIAL SKELETON. THE VERTEBRAL COLUMN IS THE DEFINING CHARACTERISTIC OF A VERTEBRATE IN WHICH THE NOTOCHORD (A FLEXIBLE ROD OF UNIFORM COMPOSITION) FOUND IN ALL CHORDATES HAS BEEN REPLACED BY A SEGMENTED SERIES OF BONE: VERTEBRAE SEPARATED BY INTERVERTEBRAL DISCS.[1] THE VERTEBRAL COLUMN HOUSES THE SPINAL CANAL, A CAVITY THAT ENCLOSES AND PROTECTS THE SPINAL CORD.

THERE ARE ABOUT 50,000 SPECIES OF ANIMALS THAT HAVE A A VERTEBRAL COLUMN. THE HUMAN VERTEBRAL COLUMN IS ONE OF THE MOST-STUDIED EXAMPLES.

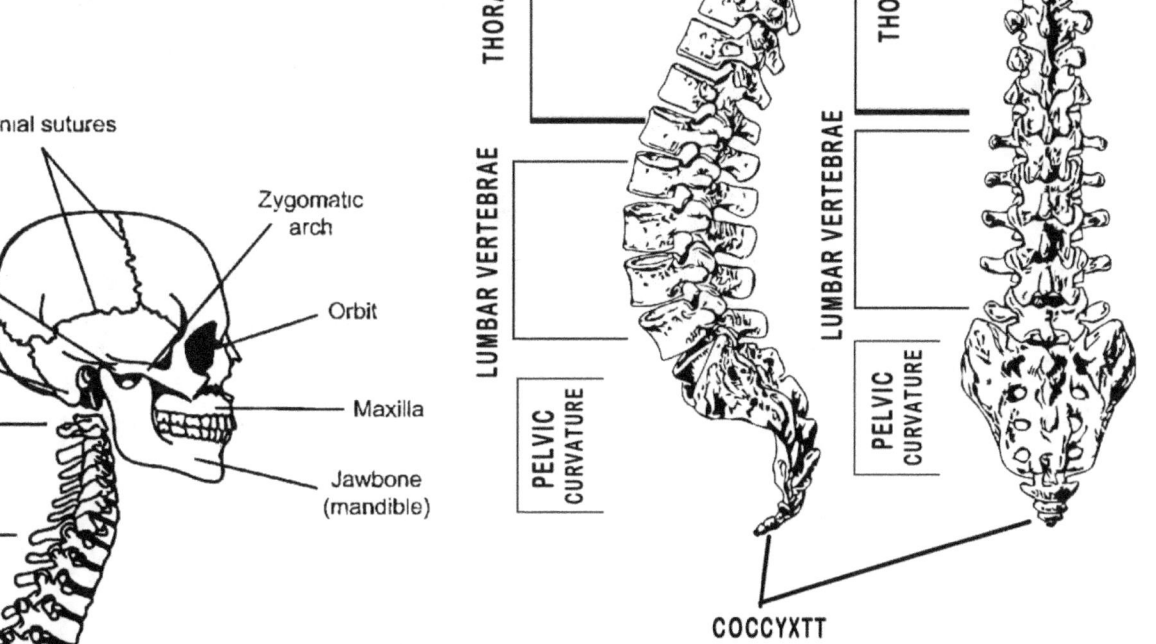

VERTEBRAE

THE VERTEBRAE IN THE HUMAN VERTEBRAL COLUMN ARE DIVIDED INTO DIFFERENT REGIONS, WHICH CORRESPOND TO THE CURVES OF THE SPINAL COLUMN. THE ARTICULATING ARE NAMED ACCORDING TO THEIR REGION OF THE SPINE. VERTEBRAE IN THESE REGIONS ARE ESSENTIALLY ALIKE, WITH MINOR VARIATION. THESE REGIONS ARE CALLED THE CERVICAL SPINE, THORACIC SPINE, LUMBAR SPINE, SACRUM, AND COCCYX. THERE ARE SEVEN CERVICAL VERTEBRAE, TWELVE THORACIC VERTEBRAE, AND FIVE LUMBAR VERTEBRAE. THE NUMBER OF VERTEBRAE IN A REGION CAN VARY BUT OVERALL THE NUMBER REMAINS THE SAME. THE NUMBER OF THOSE IN THE CERVICAL REGION, HOWEVER, IS ONLY RARELY CHANGED. THE VERTEBRAE OF THE CERVICAL, THORACIC, AND LUMBAR SPINES ARE INDEPENDENT BONES AND GENERALLY QUITE SIMILAR. THE VERTEBRAE OF THE SACRUM AND COCCYX ARE USUALLY FUSED AND UNABLE TO MOVE INDEPENDENTLY. TWO SPECIAL VERTEBRAE ARE THE ATLAS AND AXIS, ON WHICH THE HEAD RESTS.

INDIVIDUAL VERTEBRAE ARE NAMED ACCORDING TO THEIR REGION AND POSITION. FROM TOP TO BOTTOM, THE VERTEBRAE ARE:
- CERVICAL SPINE: 7 VERTEBRAE (C1-C7)
- THORACIC SPINE: 12 VERTEBRAE (T1-T12)
- LUMBAR SPINE: 5 VERTEBRAE (L1-L5)
- SACRUM: 5 (FUSED) VERTEBRAE (S1-S5)
- COCCYX: 4 (3-5) (FUSED) VERTEBRAE (TAILBONE)

AXIAL SKELETON

IS THE PART OF THE SKELETON THAT CONSISTS OF THE BONES OF THE HEAD HEAD AND TRUNK OF A VERTEBRATE. IN THE HUMAN SKELETON, IT CONSISTS OF 80 BONES AND IS COMPOSED OF SIX PARTS; THE SKULL (22 BONES), THE OSSICLES OF THE MIDDLE EAR, THE HYOID BONE, THE RIB CAGE, STERNUM AND THE VERTEBRAL COLUMN. THE AXIAL SKELETON TOGETHER WITH THE APPENDICULAR SKELETON FORM THE COMPLETE SKELETON. ANOTHER DEFINITION OF AXIAL SKELETON IS THE BONES INCLUDING THE VERTEBRAE, SACRUM, COCCYX, RIBS, AND STERNUM.

THE AXIAL SKELETON CONSISTS OF 80 BONES:

- THE SKULL, WHICH CONTAINS 22 BONES, FROM WHICH 8 ARE CRANIAL AND 14 ARE FACIAL,
- 6 MIDDLE EAR OSSICLES (3 IN EACH EAR),
- 1 HYOID BONE IN THE NECK,
- 26 BONES OF VERTEBRAL COLUMN,
- 1 CHEST BONE (STERNUM), AND
- 24 RIBS (12 PAIRS).

STRUCTURE

FLAT BONES HOUSE THE BRAIN AND OTHER VITAL ORGANS. THIS ARTICLE MAINLY DEALS WITH THE AXIAL SKELETONS OF HUMANS; HOWEVER, IT IS IMPORTANT TO UNDERSTAND THE EVOLUTIONARY LINEAGE OF THE AXIAL SKELETON. THE HUMAN AXIAL SKELETON CONSISTS OF 80 DIFFERENT BONES. IT IS THE MEDIAL CORE OF THE BODY AND CONNECTS THE PELVIS TO THE BODY, WHERE THE APPENDIX SKELETON ATTACHES. AS THE SKELETON GROWS OLDER THE BONES GET WEAKER WITH THE EXCEPTION OF THE SKULL. THE SKULL REMAINS STRONG TO PROTECT THE BRAIN FROM INJURY.

MALE PELVIS:
THE LOWER PART OF THE ABDOMEN THAT IS LOCATED BETWEEN THE HIP BONES IN A MALE. THE MALE PELVIS IS MORE ROBUST, NARROWER, AND TALLER THAN THE FEMALE PELVIS. THE ANGLE OF THE MALE PUBIC ARCH AND THE SACRUM

FEMALE PELVIS:
THE LOWER PART OF THE ABDOMEN THAT IS LOCATED BETWEEN THE HIP BONES IN A FEMALE. THE FEMALE PELVIS IS USUALLY MORE DELICATE THAN, WIDER THAN, AND NOTLOREM IPSUM AS HIGH AS THE MALE PELVIS. THE ANGLE OF THE FEMALE PUBIC ARCH IS WIDE AND ROUND. THE FEMALE SACRUM IS WIDER THAN THE MALE'S, AND THE ILIAC BONE IS FLATTER. THE PELVIC BASIN OF THE FEMALE IS MORE SPACIOUS AND LESS FUNNEL-SHAPED THAN THE MALE'S. FROM A PURELY ANATOMIC VIEWPOINT, THE FEMALE PELVIS IS BETTER SUITED THAN THE MALE PELVIS TO ACCOMMODATE A FETUS DURING PREGNANCY AND PERMIT THE BABY TO BE BORN.

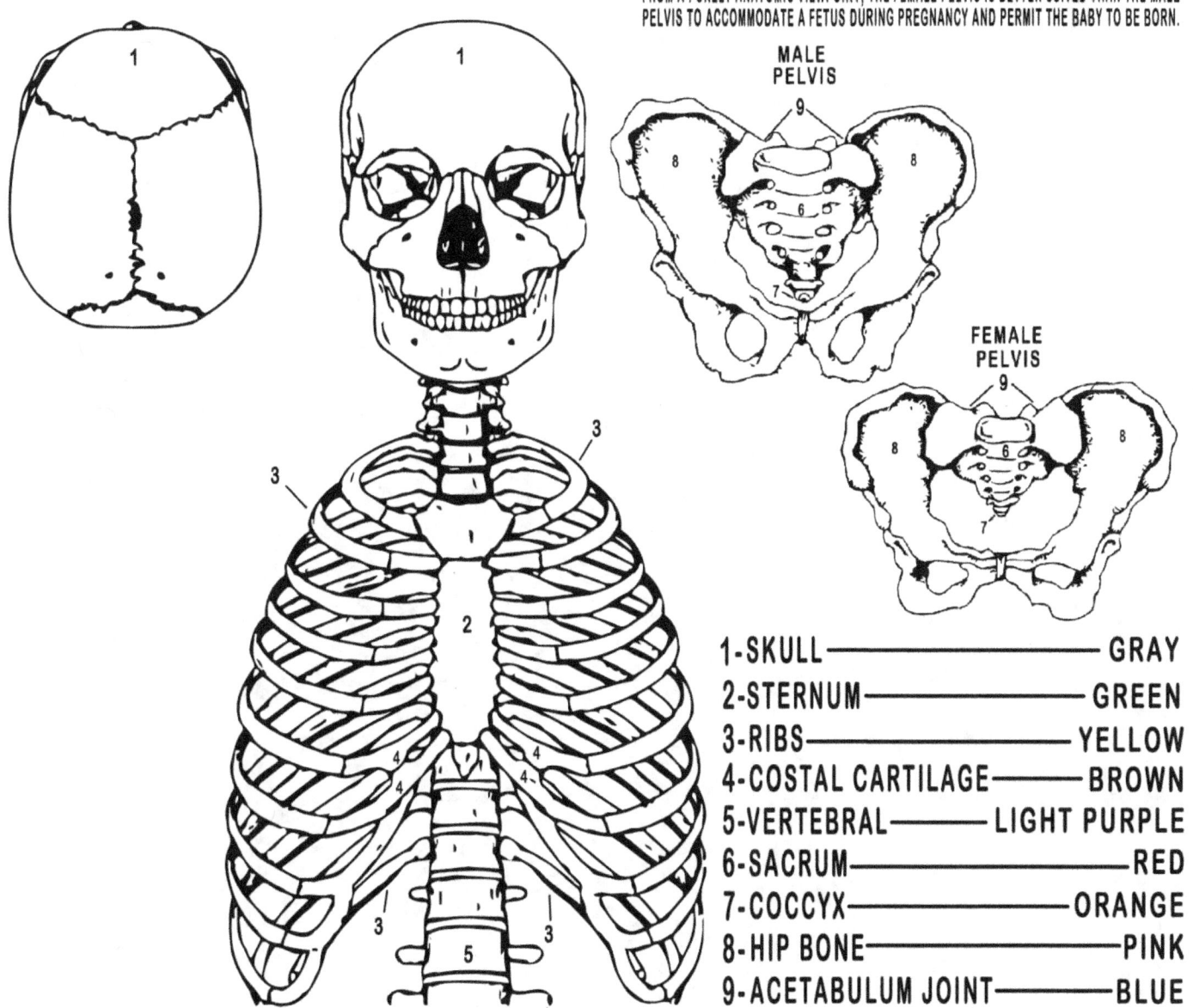

1 - SKULL —————————— GRAY
2 - STERNUM ———————— GREEN
3 - RIBS —————————— YELLOW
4 - COSTAL CARTILAGE ——— BROWN
5 - VERTEBRAL ———— LIGHT PURPLE
6 - SACRUM ——————————— RED
7 - COCCYX ———————— ORANGE
8 - HIP BONE ——————————— PINK
9 - ACETABULUM JOINT ——— BLUE

APPENDICULAR SKELETON
UPPER EXTREMITIES

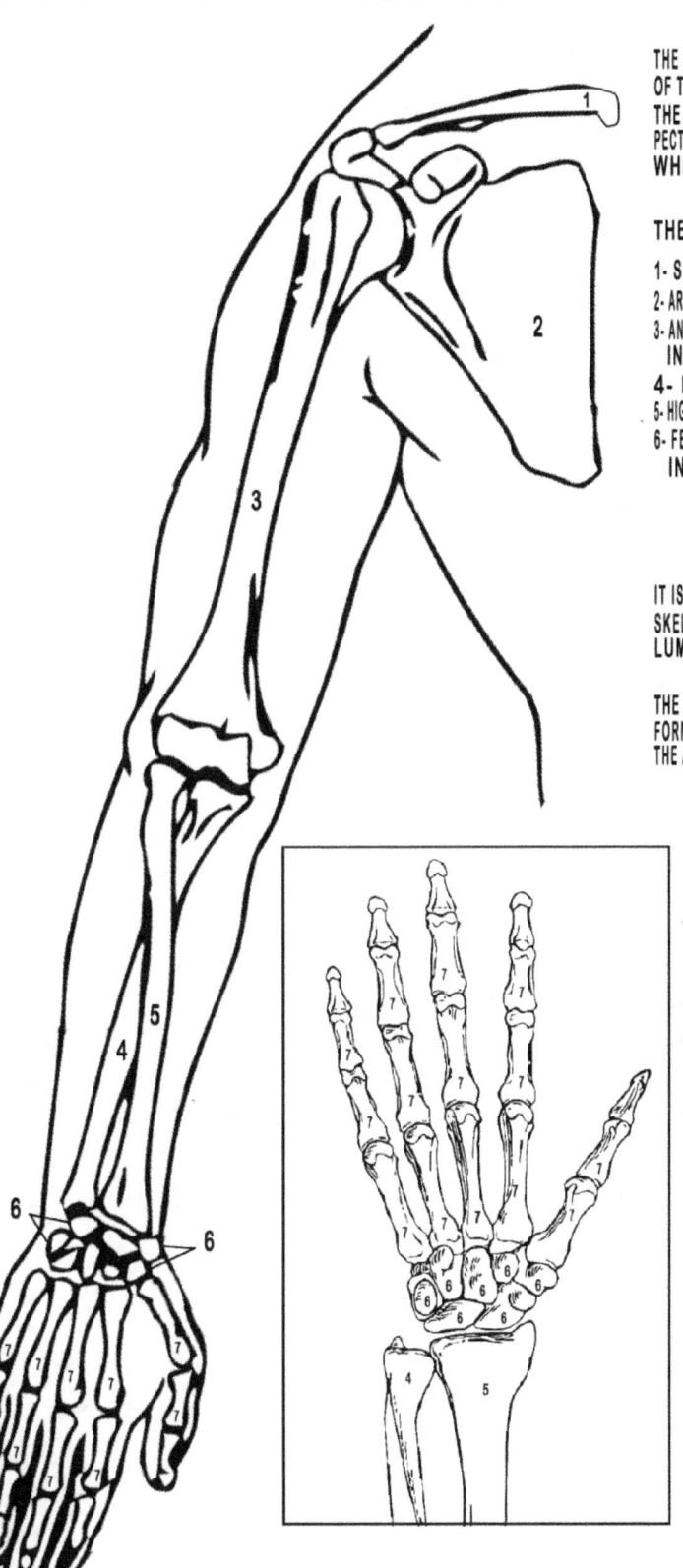

THE APPENDICULAR SKELETON IS THE PORTION OF THE SKELETON OF VERTEBRATES CONSISTING OF THE BONES THAT SUPPORT THE APPENDAGES. THE APPENDICULAR SKELETON INCLUDES THE SKELETAL ELEMENTS WITHIN THE LIMBS, AS WELL AS SUPPORTING SHOULDER GIRDLE PECTORAL AND PELVIC GIRDLE.[1] THE WORD APPENDICULAR IS THE ADJECTIVE OF THE NOUN APPENDAGE, WHICH ITSELF MEANS A PART THAT IS JOINED TO SOMETHING LARGER.

THE APPENDICULAR SKELETON IS DIVIDED INTO SIX MAJOR REGIONS:

1- SHOULDER GIRDLES (4 BONES) - LEFT AND RIGHT CLAVICLE (2) AND SCAPULA (2).
2- ARMS AND FOREARMS (6 BONES) - LEFT AND RIGHT HUMERUS (2) (ARM), ULNA (2) AND RADIUS (2) (FOREARM).
3- ANDS (54 BONES) - LEFT AND RIGHT CARPALS (16) (WRIST), METACARPALS (10), PROXIMAL PHALANGES (10), INTERMEDIATE PHALANGES (8) AND DISTAL PHALANGES (10).
4- PELVIS (6 BONES) - ILIUM (2), ISCHIUM (2) AND PUBIS (2).
5- HIGHS AND LEGS (8 BONES) - LEFT AND RIGHT FEMUR (2) (THIGH), PATELLA (2) (KNEE), TIBIA (2) AND FIBULA (2) (LEG).
6- FEET AND ANKLES (52 BONES) - LEFT AND RIGHT TARSALS (14) (ANKLE), METATARSALS (10), INTERMEDIATE PHALANGES (8) AND DISTAL PHALANGES (10).

IT IS IMPORTANT TO REALIZE THAT THROUGH ANATOMICAL VARIATION IT IS COMMON FOR THE SKELETON TO HAVE MANY ACCESSORY BONES (SUTURAL BONES IN THE SKULL, CERVICAL RIBS, LUMBAR RIBS AND EVEN EXTRA LUMBAR VERTEBRAE).

THE APPENDICULAR SKELETON OF 126 BONES AND THE AXIAL SKELETON OF 80 BONES TOGETHER FORM THE COMPLETE SKELETON OF 206 BONES IN THE HUMAN BODY. UNLIKE THE AXIAL SKELETON THE APPENDICULAR SKELETON IS UNFUSED. THIS ALLOWS FOR A MUCH GREATER RANGE OF MOTION.[2]

1- CLAVICLE —————————— GREEN
2- SCAPULA —————————— PINK
3- HUMERUS —————————— PURPLE
4- ULNA —————————————— TURQUOISE
5- RADIUS —————————————— BLUE
6- CARPAL BONES —————— LIGHT BLUE
7- PHALANGES —————————— RED

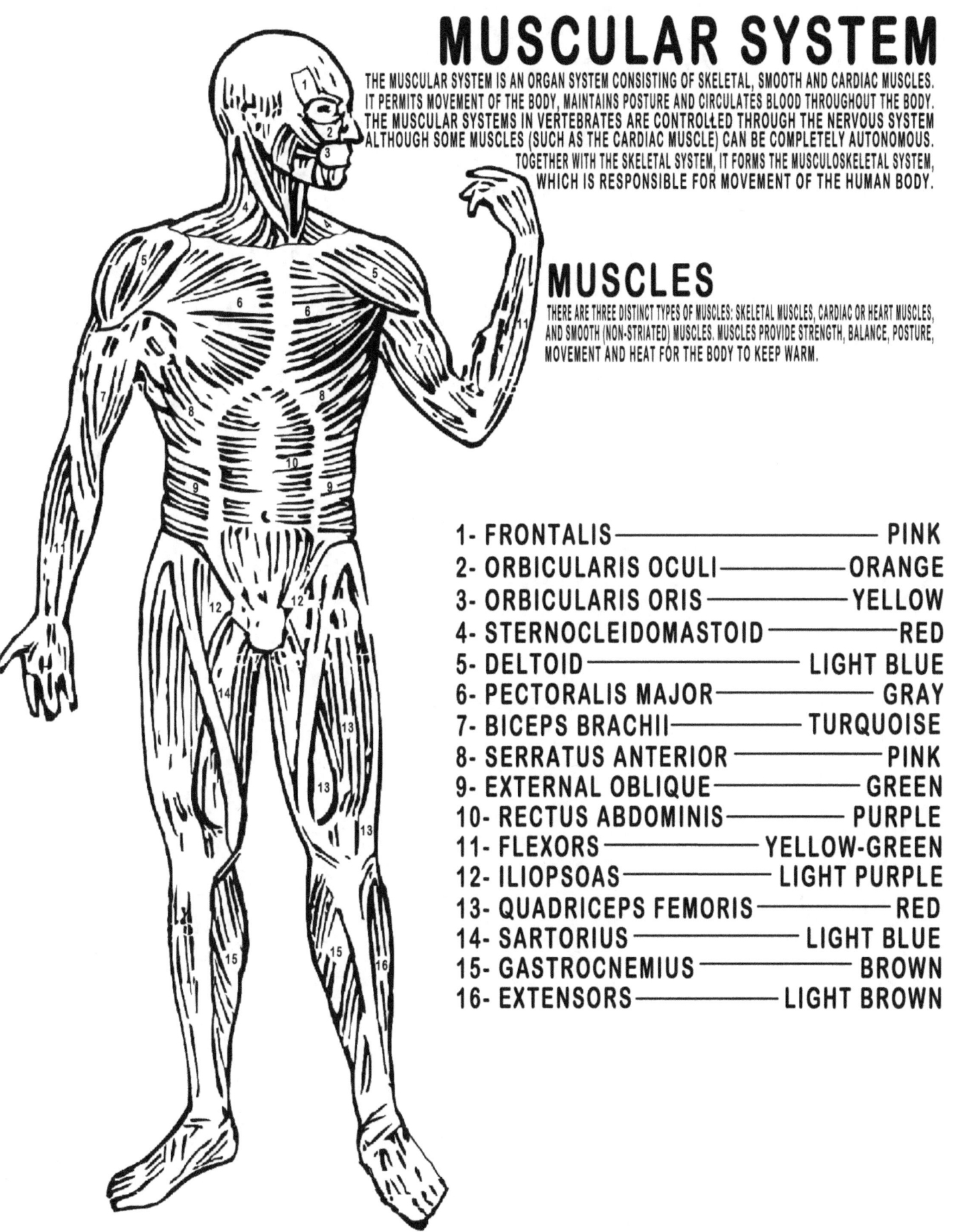

MUSCLES OF FACE, HEAD, NECK

THE FACIAL MUSCLES ARE STRIATED MUSCLES THAT ATTACH TO THE BONES OF THE SKULL TO PERFORM IMPORTANT FUNCTIONS FOR DAILY LIFE INCLUDING MASTICATION AND FACIAL EXPRESSIONS. THESE MUSCLES ARE LOCATED MEDIALLY TO THE EARS, SUPERIOR TO THELOREM IPSUM MANDIBLE, AND INFERIOR TO CORONAL SUTURE OF THE SKULL. DEFICITS IN THESE MUSCLES CAN LEAD TO SIGNIFICANT IMPAIRMENT OF DAILY FUNCTION.

THE FACIAL MUSCLES OF THE SPLANCHNOCRANIUM ACT IN SYNCHRONY. FOR EXAMPLE, DURING CHEWING THE PERIORAL FACIAL MUSCLES ARE ACTIVATED AT THE SAME TIME AS THE ORBICULARIS ORIS. DEPENDING ON THE CHEWING (RIGHT OR LEFT OR CENTRAL) AND THE CHEWED OBJECT, CHANGE THE INTERVENTION PATTERN OF THE MUSCLES OF THE ENTIRE FACE, FROM THE SUPERFICIAL MUSCLES TO THE DEEP MUSCLES. TO EMPHASIZE THIS CONCEPT AND TAKE ANOTHER EXAMPLE, THERE IS A CLOSE FASCIAL RELATIONSHIP BETWEEN THE TEMPORALIS MUSCLE AND THE BUCCINATOR MUSCLE. THE INFERIOR MUSCLE FIBRES OF THE BUCCINATOR ARISE FROM THE ANTERIOR PORTION OF THE DEEP TENDON OF THE TEMPORALIS. THE TWO MUSCLES WORK TO IMPROVE THEIR FUNCTIONS, FROM CHEWING TO THE OPENING AND MOVEMENT OF THE JAW, TO SPEECH.

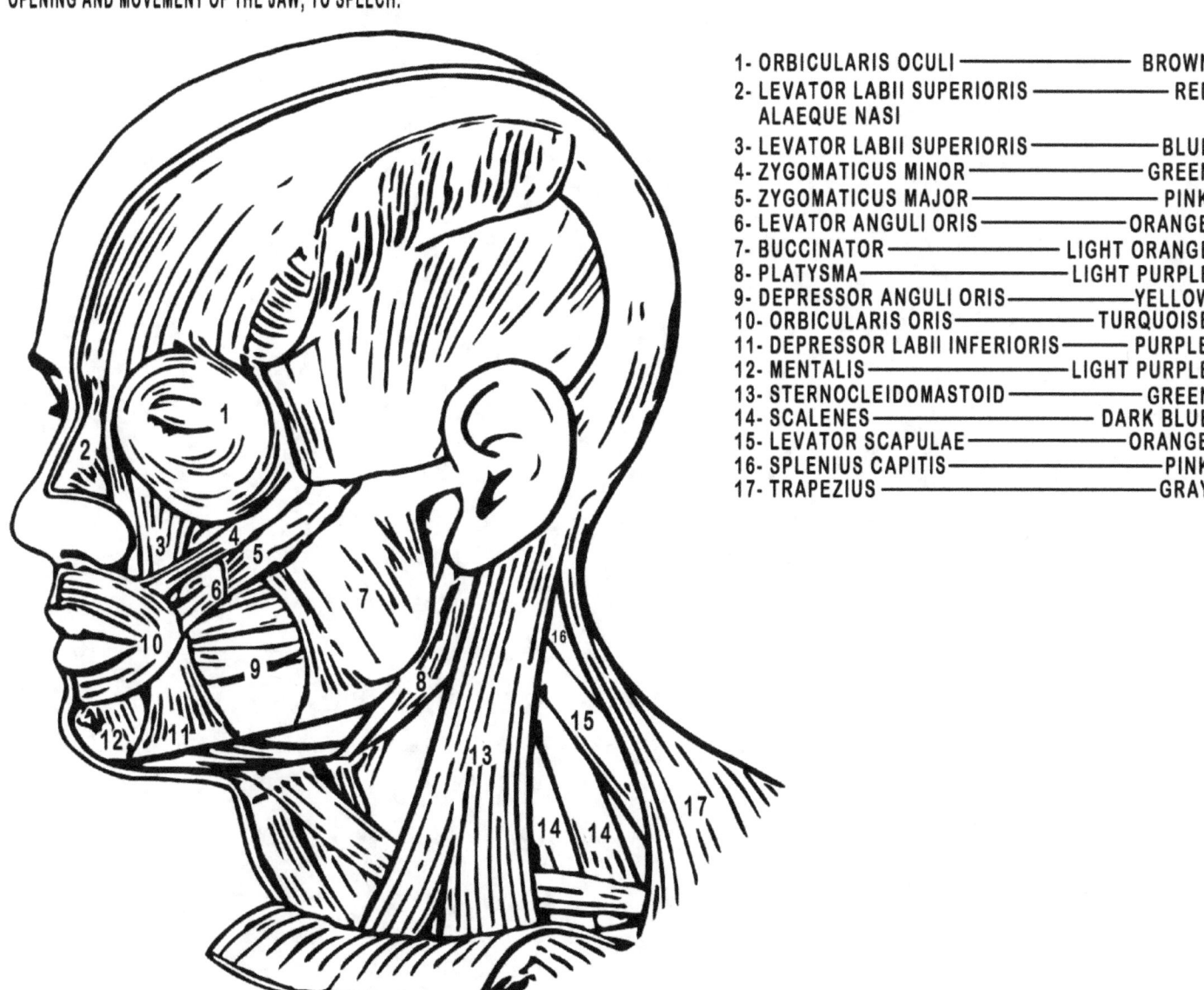

1- ORBICULARIS OCULI — BROWN
2- LEVATOR LABII SUPERIORIS ALAEQUE NASI — RED
3- LEVATOR LABII SUPERIORIS — BLUE
4- ZYGOMATICUS MINOR — GREEN
5- ZYGOMATICUS MAJOR — PINK
6- LEVATOR ANGULI ORIS — ORANGE
7- BUCCINATOR — LIGHT ORANGE
8- PLATYSMA — LIGHT PURPLE
9- DEPRESSOR ANGULI ORIS — YELLOW
10- ORBICULARIS ORIS — TURQUOISE
11- DEPRESSOR LABII INFERIORIS — PURPLE
12- MENTALIS — LIGHT PURPLE
13- STERNOCLEIDOMASTOID — GREEN
14- SCALENES — DARK BLUE
15- LEVATOR SCAPULAE — ORANGE
16- SPLENIUS CAPITIS — PINK
17- TRAPEZIUS — GRAY

MUSCLE OF THE TORSO

THE MUSCLES OF THE TORSO ARE INTERESTING ON MANY LEVELS. FIRST, UNLIKE THE MUSCLES OF THE FACIAL REGION, THEIR SHAPES ARE SOMEWHAT RECOGNIZABLE ON THE SURFACE. SECOND, SOME OF THE SUPERFICIAL MUSCLES ARE ALREADY KNOWN BY MOST PEOPLE, THOUGH MOST LIKELY BY THEIR COMMON NAMES: THE SHOULDER MUSCLE (TRAPEZIUS), THE CHEST OR PECTORAL MUSCLE (PECTORALIS MAJOR), THE "ABS" OR "SIX-PACK" (RECTUS ABDOMINIS), AND THE "FLANK PAD" OR "LOVE HANDLES" (EXTERNAL OBLIQUE). THIRD, THE MUSCLES OF THE TORSO DO NOT MOVE JUST THE TORSO (VERTEBRAL COLUMN AND RIB CAGE) BUT ALSO THE SHOULDER GIRDLE, WHICH INCLUDES THE SCAPULA BONES AND CLAVICLES, AS WELL AS THE UPPER ARMS (HUMERUS BONES). THERE ARE MANY WAYS TO CATEGORIZE THE TORSO MUSCLES. ONE WAY IS TO GROUP OF THE BODY, BUT THEY CAN ALSO BE CLASSIFIED BY ANATOMICAL REGIONS (ABDOMINAL REGION, SCAPULAR REGION, PECTORAL REGION) OR BY THEIR PLACEMENT IN RELATION TO THE SURFACE (SUPERFICIAL LAYER, INTERMEDIATE LAYER, DEEP LAYER).

FOR LEARNING PURPOSES, A COMBINATION OF SYSTEMS IS USED IN THIS CHAPTER. FIRST, LET'S LOOK AT THE TORSO MUSCLES ACCORDING TO THEIR PLACEMENT ON THE BODY FROM FRONT (ANTERIOR), BACK (POSTERIOR), AND SIDE (LATERAL) VIEWS, AS SHOWN IN THE FOLLOWING DRAWINGS.

1- DELTOID ——————— LIGHT PURPLE
2- PECTORALIS MAJOR ——————— RED
3- LATISSIMUS DORSI ——————— GREEN
4- SERRATUS ANTERIOR ——————— PINK
5- EXTERNAL OBLIQUE ——————— YELLOW
6- RECTUS ABDOMINIS ——————— BLUE
7- TERES MAJOR ——————— LIGHT BLUE
8- DORSAL ——————— TURQUOISE

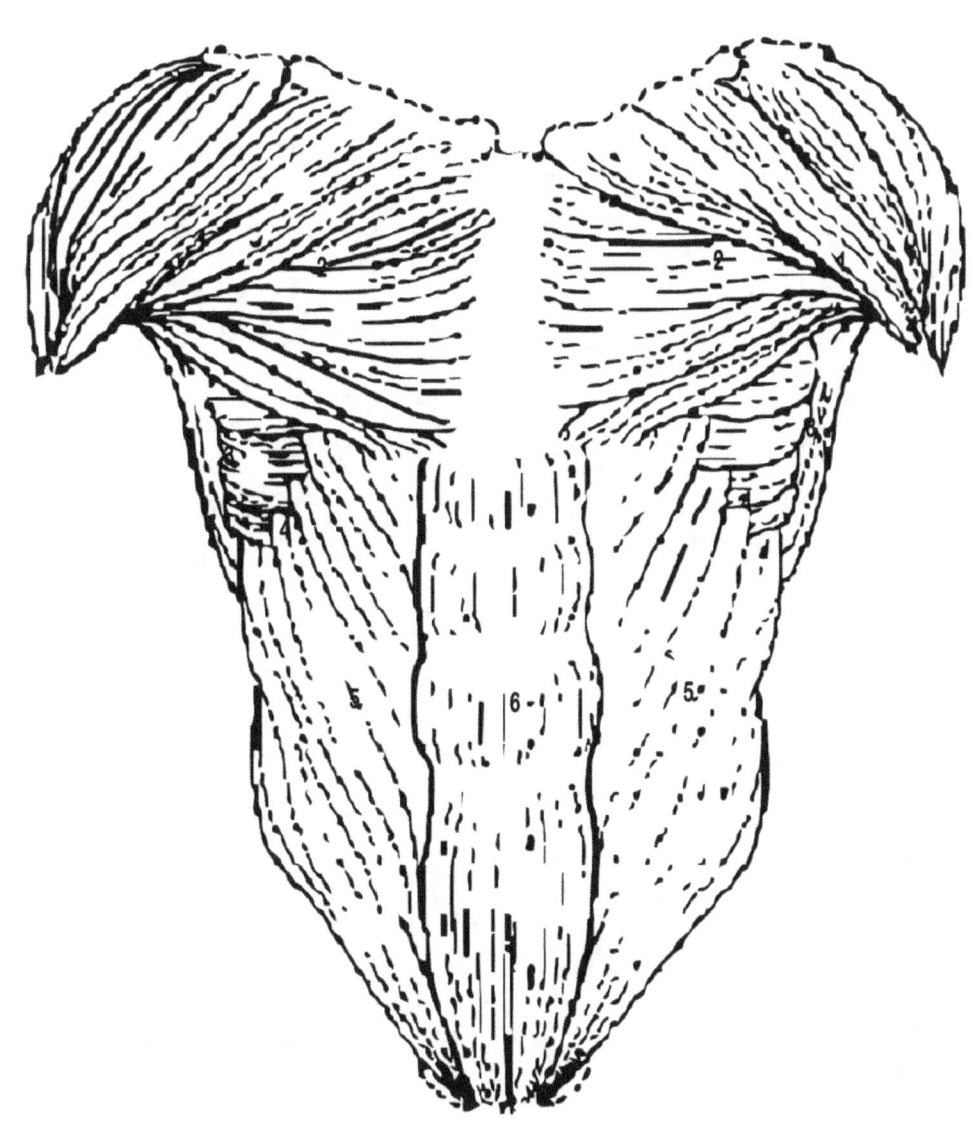

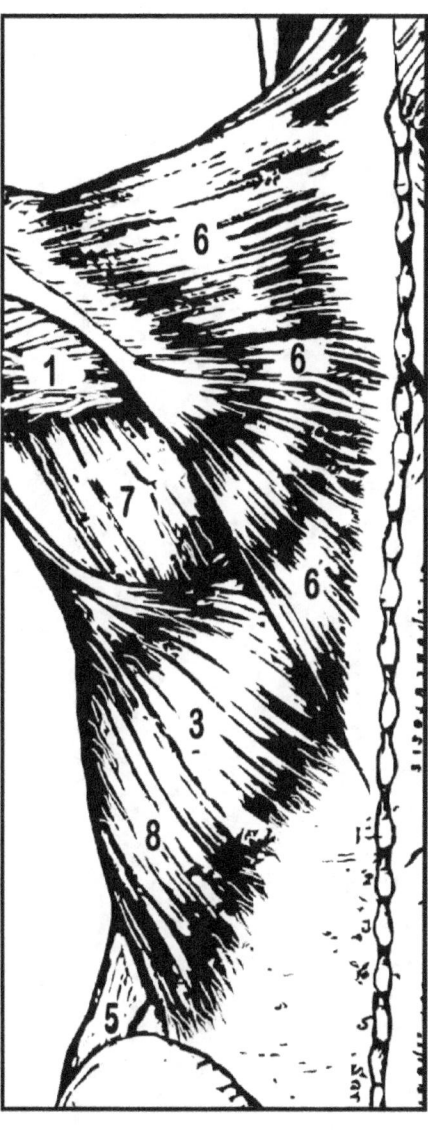

MUSCLES OF THE UPPER LIMB

THE MUSCLES OF THE UPPER LIMB CAN BE DIVIDED INTO 6 DIFFERENT REGIONS: PECTORAL, SHOULDER, UPPER ARM, ANTERIOR FOREARM, POSTERIOR FOREARM, AND THE HAND. THERE ARE 4 MUSCLES OF THE PECTORAL REGION:
PECTORALIS MAJOR, PECTORALIS MINOR, SERRATUS ANTERIOR AND SUBCLAVIUS. COLLECTIVELY, THESE MUSCLES ARE INVOLVED IN MOVEMENT AND STABILISATION OF THE SCAPULA, AS WELL AS MOVEMENTS OF THE UPPER LIMB.

THE MUSCLES OF THE SHOULDER JOINT CAN BE DIVIDED INTO AN INTRINSIC AND EXTRINSIC GROUP; THE EXTRINSIC GROUP ORIGINATE FROM THE TORSO AND ATTACH TO THE BONES OF THE SHOULDER, WHEREAS THE INTRINSIC ONES ORIGINATE FROM THE BONES OF THE SHOULDER AND ATTACH THE HUMERUS. THEY COLLECTIVELY ACT TO MOVE THE UPPER ARM AND STABILISE THE SHOULDER JOINT.

THE UPPER ARM, LOCATED BETWEEN THE SHOULDER AND ELBOW JOINT, HAS AN ANTERIOR AND POSTERIOR COMPARTMENT. THE MUSCLES LOCATED IN THE ANTERIOR COMPARTMENT ARE INVOLVED IN FLEXION AT THE ELBOW AND SHOULDER JOINT WHEREAS MUSCLE IN THE POSTERIOR COMPARTMENT, TRICEPS BRACHII, EXTENDS THE ARM AT THE ELBOW JOINT.

THE MUSCLES OF THE FOREARM ARE SUBDIVIDED INTO AN ANTERIOR AND POSTERIOR COMPARTMENT. THE MUSCLES OF THE ANTERIOR COMPARTMENT ARE FURTHER DIVIDED INTO A SUPERFICIAL, INTERMEDIATE AND DEEP LAYER; INNERVATED BY BOTH THE ULNAR AND MEDIAN NERVE, THEY COLLECTIVELY ACT TO PRONATE THE FOREARM AND TO FLEX THE WRIST AND THE DIGITS.

THE MUSCLES OF THE POSTERIOR COMPARTMENT ARE SEPARATED INTO A SUPERFICIAL AND DEEP LAYER. THESE MUSCLES ARE INNERVATED BY THE RADIAL NERVE AND ARE KNOWN AS THE EXTENSOR MUSCLES DUE TO THEIR GENERAL ACTION OF EXTENDING THE WRIST AND THE DIGITS.

THE MUSCLES OF THE HAND CAN BE DIVIDED INTO AN EXTRINSIC AND INTRINSIC GROUP. THE EXTRINSIC GROUP ORIGINATE FROM THE FOREARM AND ATTACH TO THE BONES OF THE HAND, THEY ARE ASSOCIATED WITH FORCEFUL OR NON-PRECISE MOVEMENTS. ON THE OTHER HAND, THE INTRINSIC GROUP ORIGINATE AND ATTACH WITHIN THE HAND ITSELF AND ARE MORE INVOLVED WITH FINE-TUNED AND DELICATE MOVEMENTS. BOTH GROUPS ARE INNERVATED BY THE ULNAR AND MEDIAN NERVE.

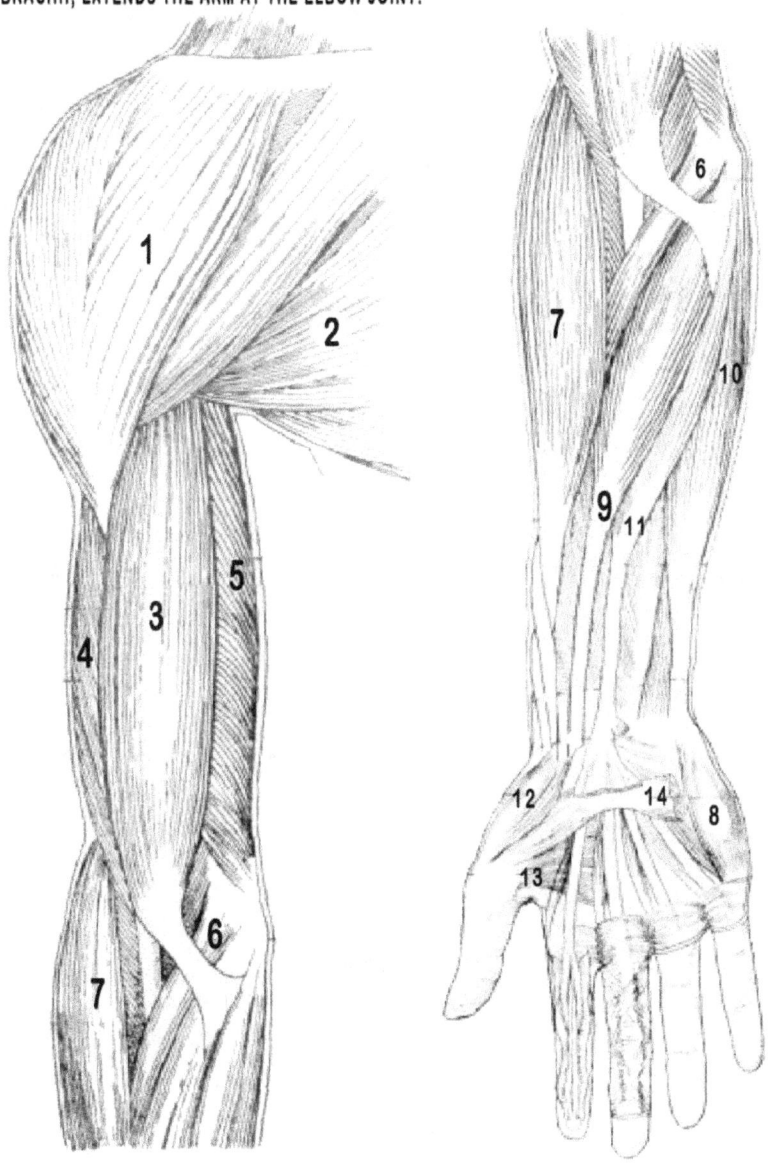

1- DELTOID — PINK
2- PECTORALIS MAJOR — YELLOW
3- BICEPS — LIGHT PURPLE
4- BRACHIALIS ANTICUS — GRAY
5- LONG-HEAD OF BICEPS — RED
6- PRONATOR RADII TERES — GREEN
7- SUPINATOR LONGUS — PURPLE
8- ABDUCTOR MINIMI DIGITI — TURQUOISE
9- FLEXOR CARPI RADIALIS — BLUE
10- FLEXOR CARPI ULNARIS — PINK
11- PALMARIS LONGUS — LIGHT BLUE
12- ABDUCTOR POLLICIS — YELLOW
13- ADDUCTOR POLLICIS — BROWN
14- PALMARIS BREVIS — LIGHT BROWN

MUSCLES OF THE LOWER LIMPS

THERE ARE FOUR MUSCLES IN THE ANTERIOR COMPARTMENT OF THE LEG; TIBIALIS ANTERIOR, EXTENSOR DIGITORUM LONGUS, EXTENSOR HALLUCIS LONGUS AND FIBULARIS TERTIUS.

COLLECTIVELY, THEY ACT TO DORSIFLEX AND INVERT THE FOOT AT THE ANKLE JOINT. THE EXTENSOR DIGITORUM LONGUS AND EXTENSOR HALLUCIS LONGUS ALSO EXTEND THE TOES. THE MUSCLES IN THIS COMPARTMENT ARE INNERVATED BY THE DEEP FIBULAR NERVE (L4-S1), AND BLOOD IS SUPPLIED VIA THE ANTERIOR TIBIAL ARTERY.

IN THIS ARTICLE, WE SHALL LOOK AT THE ACTIONS, ATTACHMENTS AND INNERVATION OF THE MUSCLES IN THE ANTERIOR COMPARTMENT OF THE LEG.

THERE ARE TWO MUSCLES IN THE LATERAL COMPARTMENT OF THE LEG; THE FIBULARIS LONGUS AND BREVIS (ALSO KNOWN AS PERONEAL LONGUS AND BREVIS). THE COMMON FUNCTION OF THE MUSCLES IS EVERSION - TURNING THE SOLE OF THE FOOT OUTWARDS. THEY ARE BOTH INNERVATED BY THE SUPERFICIAL FIBULAR NERVE.

IN THIS ARTICLE, WE SHALL LOOK AT THE ANATOMY OF THE MUSCLES IN THE LATERAL COMPARTMENT OF THE LEG - THEIR ATTACHMENTS, INNERVATION AND ACTIONS.

THE POSTERIOR COMPARTMENT OF THE LEG CONTAINS SEVEN MUSCLES, ORGANISED INTO TWO LAYERS - SUPERFICIAL AND DEEP. THE TWO LAYERS ARE SEPARATED BY A BAND OF FASCIA. THE POSTERIOR LEG IS THE LARGEST OF THE THREE COMPARTMENTS. COLLECTIVELY, THE MUSCLES IN THIS AREA PLANTARFLEX AND INVERT THE FOOT. THEY ARE INNERVATED BY THE TIBIAL NERVE, A TERMINAL BRANCH OF THE SCIATIC NERVE.

IN THIS ARTICLE, WE SHALL LOOK AT THE ATTACHMENTS, ACTIONS AND INNERVATION OF THE MUSCLES IN THE POSTERIOR COMPARTMENT OF THE LEG.

1- A. GLUTEUS MEDIUS AND B. MAXIMUS —— PURPLE
2- TENSOR FASCIAE LATAE —— YELLOW
3- SARTORIUS —— YELLOW-GREEN
4- PECTINEUS —— GRAY
5- ADDUCTOR LONGUS —— LIGHT GREEN
6- GRACILIS —— PINK
7- A. VASTUS LATERALIS AND B. MEDIALIS —— RED
8- RECTUS FEMORIS —— LIGHT BLUE
9- GASTROCNEMIUS —— GREEN
10- SOLEUS —— ORANGE
11- PERONEUS —— BLUE
12- TIBIALIS ANTERIOR —— BROWN
13- A. TENDONS AND B. TENDOCALCANEUS —— YELLOW
AND C. TENDON OF QUADRICEPS FEMORIS
14- A. SEMIMEMBRANOSUS AND —— TURQUOISE
B. SEMITENDINOSUS
15- BICEPS FEMORIS —— LIGHT BROWN
16- EXTENSOR DIGITORUM BREVIS —— LIGHT PURPLE
17- ABDUCTOR DIGITI MINIMI —— DARK BLUE
18- ABDUCTOR HALLUCIS —— DARK GREEN
19- FLEXOR DIGITORUM BREVIS —— LIGHT ORANGE

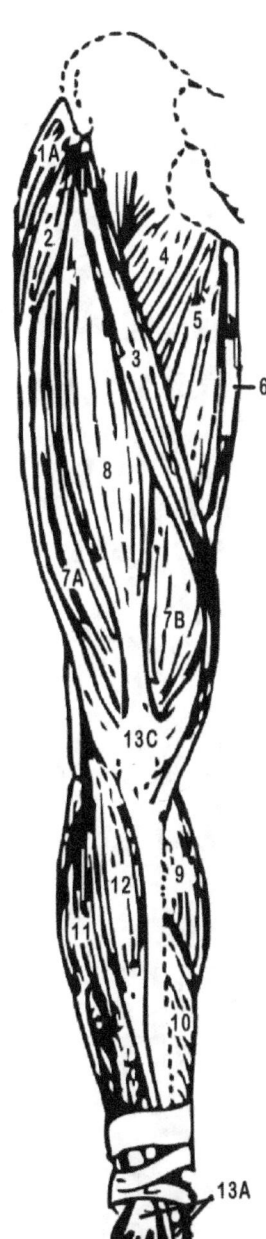
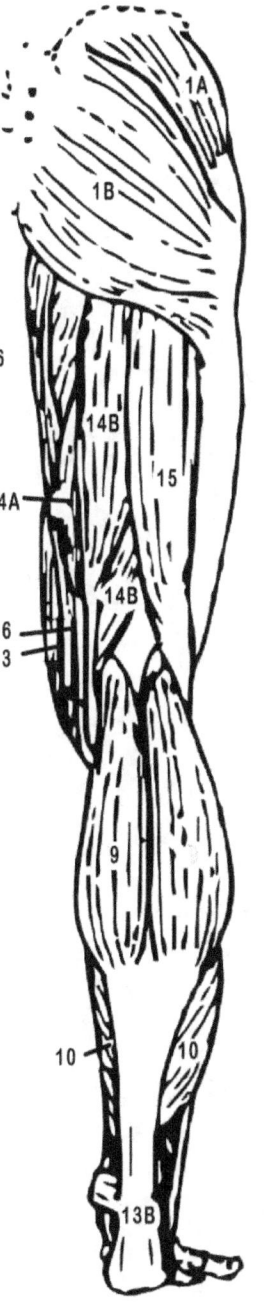

CIRCULATORY SYSTEM

THE CIRCULATORY SYSTEM, ALSO CALLED THE CARDIOVASCULAR SYSTEM OR THE VASCULAR SYSTEM, IS AN ORGAN SYSTEM THAT PERMITS BLOOD TO CIRCULATE AND TRANSPORT NUTRIENTS (SUCH AS AMINO ACIDS AND ELECTROLYTES), OXYGEN, CARBON DIOXIDE, HORMONES, AND BLOOD CELLS TO AND FROM THE CELLS IN THE BODY TO PROVIDE NOURISHMENT AND HELP IN FIGHTING DISEASES, STABILIZE TEMPERATURE AND PH, AND MAINTAIN HOMEOSTASIS.

THE CIRCULATORY SYSTEM INCLUDES THE LYMPHATIC SYSTEM, WHICH CIRCULATES LYMPH. THE PASSAGE OF LYMPH TAKES MUCH LONGER THAN THAT OF BLOOD. BLOOD IS A FLUID CONSISTING OF PLASMA, RED BLOOD CELLS, WHITE BLOOD CELLS, AND PLATELETS THAT IS CIRCULATED BY THE HEART THROUGH THE VERTEBRATE VASCULAR SYSTEM, CARRYING OXYGEN AND NUTRIENTS TO AND WASTE MATERIALS AWAY FROM ALL BODY TISSUES. LYMPH IS ESSENTIALLY RECYCLED EXCESS BLOOD PLASMA AFTER IT HAS BEEN FILTERED FROM THE INTERSTITIAL FLUID (BETWEEN CELLS) AND RETURNED TO THE LYMPHATIC SYSTEM. THE CARDIOVASCULAR (FROM LATIN WORDS MEANING "HEART" AND "VESSEL") SYSTEM COMPRISES THE BLOOD, HEART, AND BLOOD VESSELS. THE LYMPH, LYMPH NODES, AND LYMPH VESSELS FORM THE LYMPHATIC SYSTEM, WHICH RETURNS FILTERED BLOOD PLASMA FROM THE INTERSTITIAL FLUID (BETWEEN CELLS) AS LYMPH.

THE CIRCULATORY SYSTEM OF THE BLOOD IS SEEN AS HAVING TWO COMPONENTS, A SYSTEMIC CIRCULATION AND A PULMONARY CIRCULATION. WHILE HUMANS, AS WELL AS OTHER VERTEBRATES, HAVE A CLOSED CARDIOVASCULAR SYSTEM (MEANING THAT THE BLOOD NEVER LEAVES THE NETWORK OF ARTERIES, VEINS AND CAPILLARIES), SOME INVERTEBRATE GROUPS HAVE AN OPEN CARDIOVASCULAR SYSTEM. THE LYMPHATIC SYSTEM, ON THE OTHER HAND, IS AN OPEN SYSTEM PROVIDING AN ACCESSORY ROUTE FOR EXCESS INTERSTITIAL FLUID TO BE RETURNED TO THE BLOOD. THE MORE PRIMITIVE, DIPLOBLASTIC ANIMAL PHYLA LACK CIRCULATORY SYSTEMS.

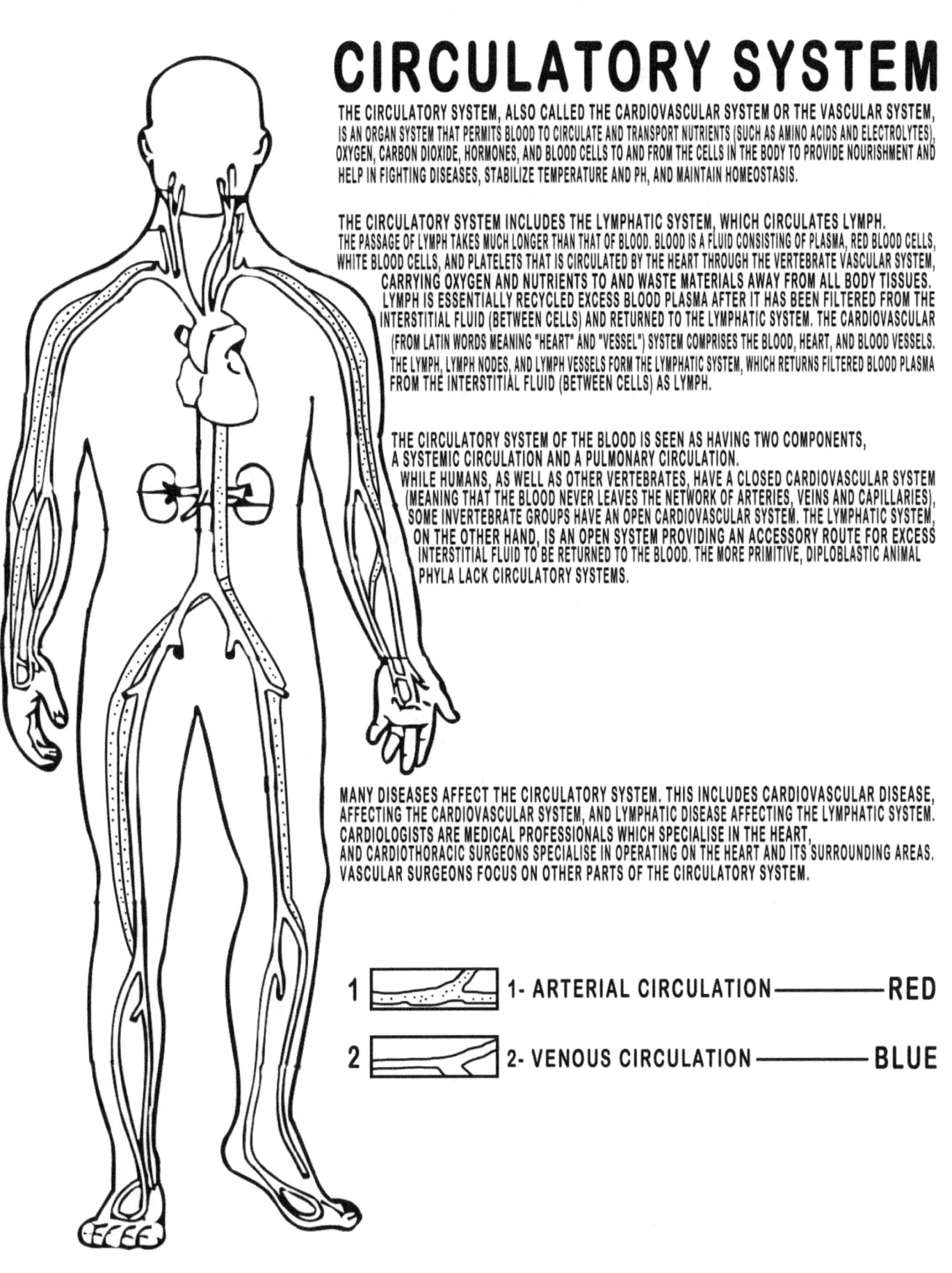

MANY DISEASES AFFECT THE CIRCULATORY SYSTEM. THIS INCLUDES CARDIOVASCULAR DISEASE, AFFECTING THE CARDIOVASCULAR SYSTEM, AND LYMPHATIC DISEASE AFFECTING THE LYMPHATIC SYSTEM. CARDIOLOGISTS ARE MEDICAL PROFESSIONALS WHICH SPECIALISE IN THE HEART, AND CARDIOTHORACIC SURGEONS SPECIALISE IN OPERATING ON THE HEART AND ITS SURROUNDING AREAS. VASCULAR SURGEONS FOCUS ON OTHER PARTS OF THE CIRCULATORY SYSTEM.

1- ARTERIAL CIRCULATION————RED

2- VENOUS CIRCULATION————BLUE

Immune System

The immune system is a network of cells, tissues and organs that defend the body against harmful toxins and microorganisms.

1. red bone marrow: *spongy tissue of the bone that produces cells of the immune system including lymphocytes and macrophages. Lymphocytes recognize antigens (harmful foreign bodies), and macrophages engulf and destroy antigens.*

2. lymphatic system: *network of lymph nodes and lymph vessels that store and transport disease-fighting immune cells.*

3. thymus: *organ of the immune system that produces a special kind of white blood cell called T-lymphocytes or T-cells. T-cells detect and destroy infected cells in the body.*

4. spleen: *lymphoid organ that contains disease-fighting white blood cells and filters the blood by destroying old blood cells and removing small particles.*

5. pharyngeal tonsils (adenoids): *lymphoid tissue located at the back of the nasal cavity thought to be the first line of defense against inhaled pathogens (harmful microorganisms).*

6. palatine tonsils: *lymphoid tissue located at the back of the throat thought to be the first line of defense against inhaled pathogens (harmful microorganisms).*

1- RED BONE MARROW ———— RED
2- LYMPHATIC SYSTEM ———— BROWN
3- THYMUS ———— GREEN
4- SPLEEN ———— DARK GREEN
5- PHARYNGEAL TONSILS ———— PINK
6- PALATINE TONSILS ———— LIGHT BLUE

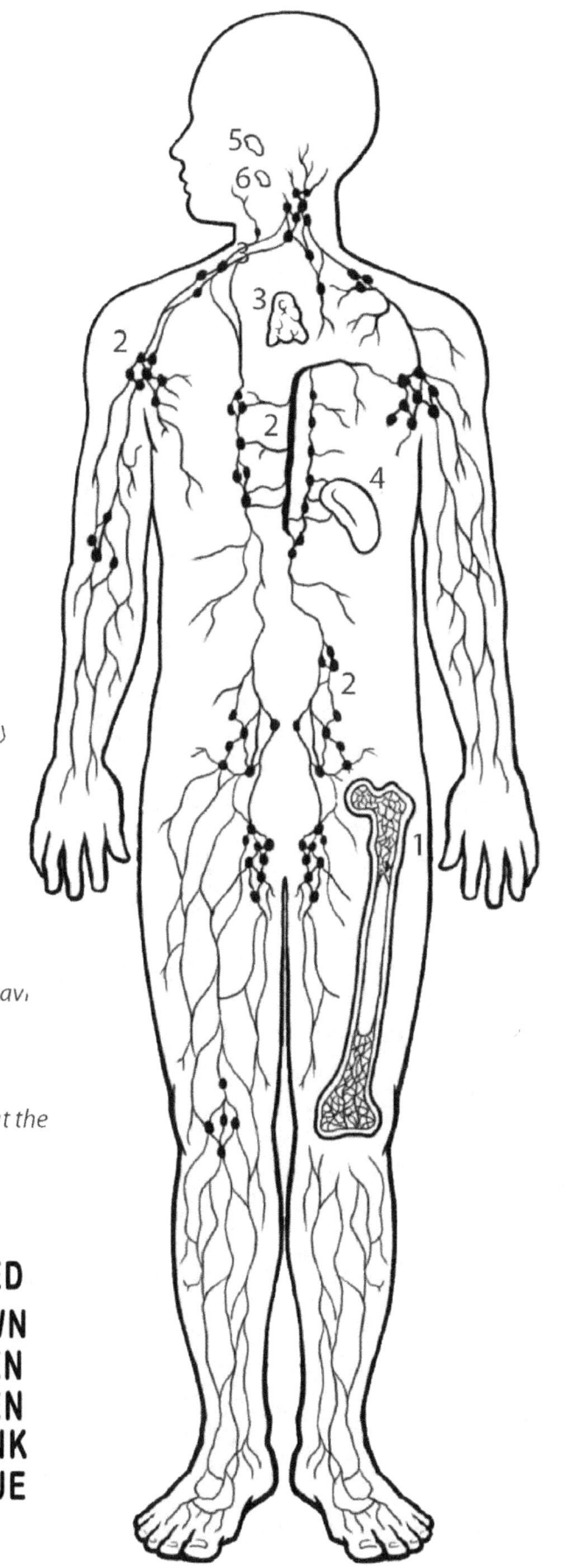

HEART

THE HEART IS A MUSCULAR ORGAN IN MOST ANIMALS, WHICH PUMPS BLOOD THROUGH THE BLOOD VESSELS OF THE CIRCULATORY SYSTEM. THE PUMPED BLOOD CARRIES OXYGEN AND NUTRIENTS TO THE BODY, WHILE CARRYING METABOLIC WASTE SUCH AS CARBON DIOXIDE TO THE LUNGS. IN HUMANS, THE HEART IS APPROXIMATELY THE SIZE OF A CLOSED FIST AND IS LOCATED BETWEEN THE LUNGS, IN THE MIDDLE COMPARTMENT OF THE CHEST.

IN HUMANS, OTHER MAMMALS, AND BIRDS, THE HEART IS DIVIDED INTO FOUR CHAMBERS: UPPER LEFT AND RIGHT ATRIA AND LOWER LEFT AND RIGHT VENTRICLES. COMMONLY THE RIGHT ATRIUM AND VENTRICLE ARE REFERRED TOGETHER AS THE RIGHT HEART AND THEIR LEFT COUNTERPARTS AS THE LEFT HEART. FISH, IN CONTRAST, HAVE TWO CHAMBERS, AN ATRIUM AND A VENTRICLE, WHILE REPTILES HAVE THREE CHAMBERS. IN A HEALTHY HEART BLOOD FLOWS ONE WAY THROUGH THE HEART DUE TO HEART VALVES, WHICH PREVENT BACKFLOW. THE HEART IS ENCLOSED IN A PROTECTIVE SAC, THE PERICARDIUM, WHICH ALSO CONTAINS A SMALL AMOUNT OF FLUID. THE WALL OF THE HEART IS MADE UP OF THREE LAYERS: EPICARDIUM, MYOCARDIUM, AND ENDOCARDIUM.

THE HEART PUMPS BLOOD WITH A RHYTHM DETERMINED BY A GROUP OF PACEMAKING CELLS IN THE SINOATRIAL NODE. THESE GENERATE A CURRENT THAT CAUSES CONTRACTION OF THE HEART, TRAVELING THROUGH THE ATRIOVENTRICULAR NODE AND ALONG THE CONDUCTION SYSTEM OF THE HEART. THE HEART RECEIVES BLOOD LOW IN OXYGEN FROM THE SYSTEMIC CIRCULATION, WHICH ENTERS THE RIGHT ATRIUM FROM THE SUPERIOR AND INFERIOR VENAE CAVAE AND PASSES TO THE RIGHT VENTRICLE. FROM HERE IT IS PUMPED INTO THE PULMONARY CIRCULATION, THROUGH THE LUNGS WHERE IT RECEIVES OXYGEN AND GIVES OFF CARBON DIOXIDE. OXYGENATED BLOOD THEN RETURNS TO THE LEFT ATRIUM, PASSES THROUGH THE LEFT VENTRICLE AND IS PUMPED OUT THROUGH THE AORTA TO THE SYSTEMIC CIRCULATION-WHERE THE OXYGEN IS USED AND METABOLIZED TO CARBON DIOXIDE. THE HEART BEATS AT A RESTING RATE CLOSE TO 72 BEATS PER MINUTE. EXERCISE TEMPORARILY INCREASES THE RATE, BUT LOWERS RESTING HEART RATE IN THE LONG TERM, AND IS GOOD FOR HEART HEALTH.

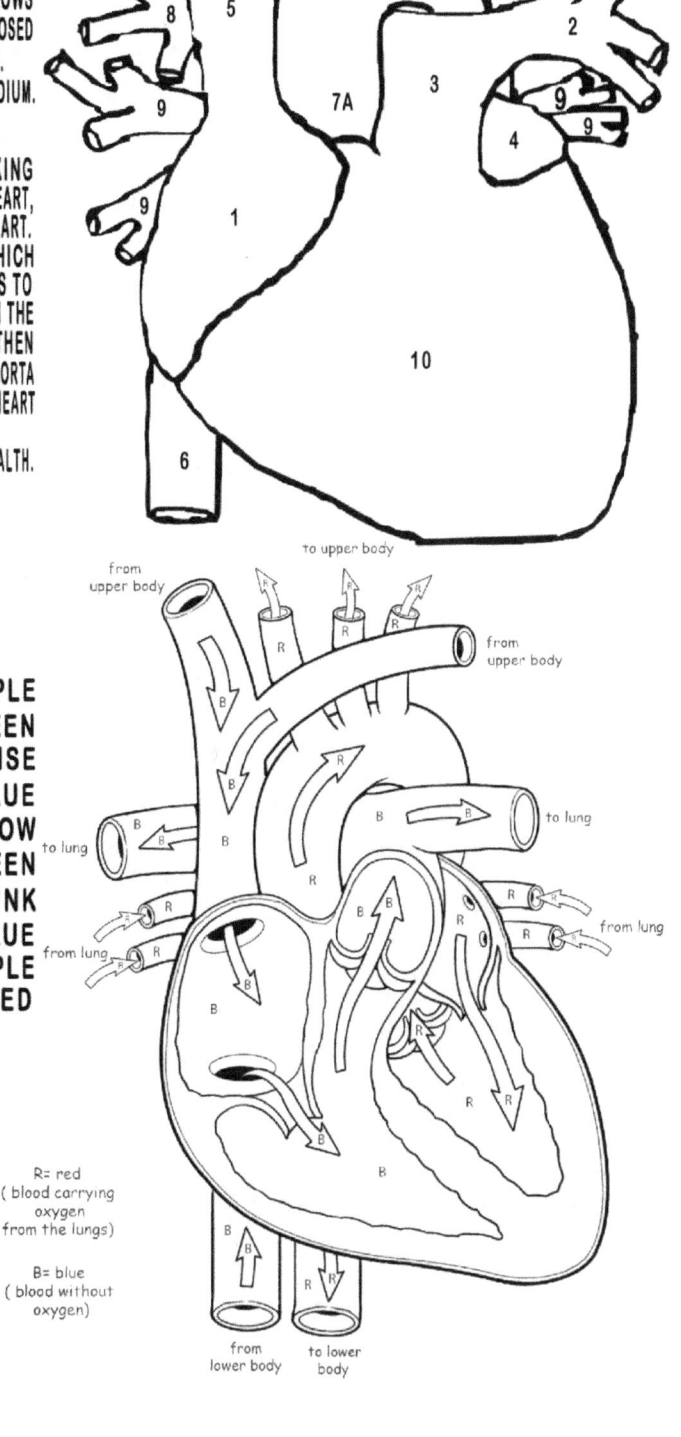

1- RIGHT ATRIUM —————————————— LIGHT PURPLE
2- RIGHT VENTRICLE ————————————— DARK GREEN
3- LEFT VENTRICLE ——————————————— TURQUOISE
4- LEFT ATRIUM ——————————————————— BLUE
5- SUPERIOR VENA CAVA ——————————— YELLOW
6- INFERIOR VENA CAVA ———————————— GREEN
7- A. ASCENDING AORTA AND B. AORTIC ARCH —— PINK
8- PULMONARY ARTERY ————————————— LIGHT BLUE
9- PULMONARY VEIN —————————————————— PURPLE
10- HEART —————————————————————————— RED

DIGESTIVE SYSTEM

THE HUMAN DIGESTIVE SYSTEM CONSISTS OF THE GASTROINTESTINAL TRACT PLUS THE ACCESSORY ORGANS OF DIGESTION (THE TONGUE, SALIVARY GLANDS, PANCREAS, LIVER, AND GALLBLADDER). DIGESTION INVOLVES THE BREAKDOWN OF FOOD INTO SMALLER AND SMALLER COMPONENTS, UNTIL THEY CAN BE ABSORBED AND ASSIMILATED INTO THE BODY. THE PROCESS OF DIGESTION HAS THREE STAGES. THE FIRST STAGE IS THE CEPHALIC PHASE OF DIGESTION WHICH BEGINS WITH GASTRIC SECRETIONS IN RESPONSE TO THE SIGHT AND SMELL OF FOOD. THIS STAGE INCLUDES THE MECHANICAL BREAKDOWN OF FOOD BY CHEWING, AND THE CHEMICAL BREAKDOWN BY DIGESTIVE ENZYMES, THAT TAKES PLACE IN THE MOUTH. SALIVA CONTAINS DIGESTIVE ENZYMES CALLED AMYLASE, AND LINGUAL LIPASE, SECRETED BY THE SALIVARY GLANDS AND SEROUS GLANDS ON THE TONGUE. THE ENZYMES START TO BREAK DOWN THE FOOD IN THE MOUTH. CHEWING, IN WHICH THE FOOD IS MIXED WITH SALIVA, BEGINS THE MECHANICAL PROCESS OF DIGESTION. THIS PRODUCES A BOLUS WHICH CAN BE SWALLOWED DOWN THE ESOPHAGUS TO ENTER THE STOMACH. IN THE STOMACH THE GASTRIC PHASE OF DIGESTION TAKES PLACE. THE FOOD IS FURTHER BROKEN DOWN BY MIXING WITH GASTRIC ACID UNTIL IT PASSES INTO THE DUODENUM, IN THE THIRD INTESTINAL PHASE OF DIGESTION

1- MOUTH — BLUE
2- SALIVARY GLAND — YELLOW
3- ESOPHAGUS — LIGHT PURPLE
4- LIVER — GREEN
5- STOMACH — GRAY
6- GALLBLADDER — LIGHT BLUE
7- PANCREAS — DARK GREEN
8- LARGE INTESTINE — PINK
9- SMALL INTESTINE — RED
10- APPENDIX — PURPLE
11- RECTUM — ORANGE
12- ANUS — TURQUOISE

RESPIRATORY SYSTEM

THE CELLS OF THE HUMAN BODY REQUIRE A CONSTANT STREAM OF OXYGEN TO STAY ALIVE. THE RESPIRATORY SYSTEM PROVIDES OXYGEN TO THE BODY'S CELLS WHILE REMOVING CARBON DIOXIDE, A WASTE PRODUCT THAT CAN BE LETHAL IF ALLOWED TO ACCUMULATE. THERE ARE 3 MAJOR PARTS OF THE RESPIRATORY SYSTEM: THE AIRWAY, THE LUNGS, AND THE MUSCLES OF RESPIRATION. THE AIRWAY, WHICH INCLUDES THE NOSE, MOUTH, PHARYNX, LARYNX, TRACHEA, BRONCHI, AND BRONCHIOLES, CARRIES AIR BETWEEN THE LUNGS AND THE BODY'S EXTERIOR.

CHOOSE YOUR OWN COLORS

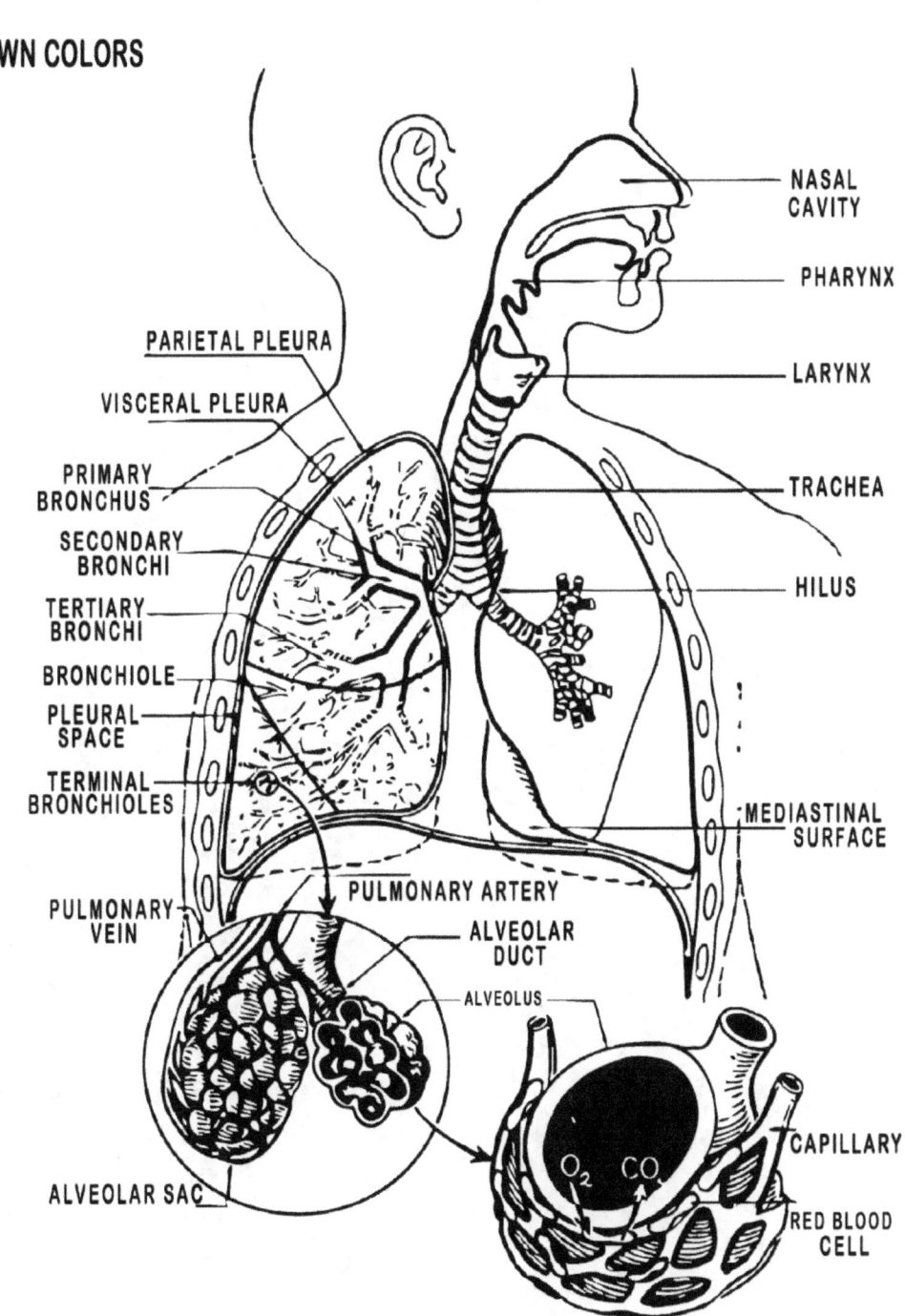

ARTERIES

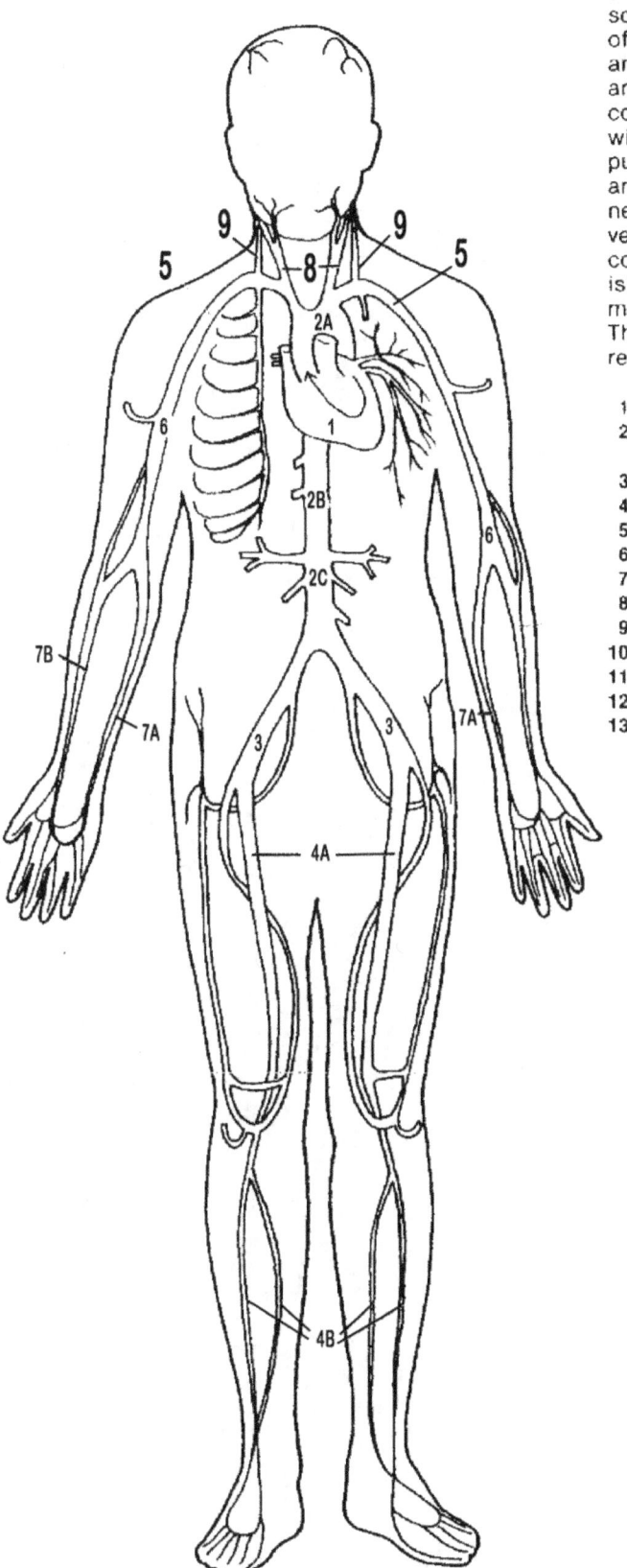

The arteries carry blood from the heart to the capillaries, dividing and then subdividing on the way until they become smaller and smaller and more and more numerous, and end in the *capillary beds* located in the body tissues. The *aorta* is the first and largest of the arteries. Adults have about seven thousand square miles of capillaries. If laid end to end, all the elements of the *vascular* (blood vessel) *system* — arteries, capillaries, and veins — would extend about seventy thousand miles. The arteries have three layers — muscle tissue, elastic fibers, and connective tissue — and expand and contract in coordination with the flow of blood passing through them. Each heartbeat pushes blood into the arteries, which expand to hold the blood and then contract behind it as the heart pumps the blood to the next section of the vascular system. The arteries' structure prevents them from collapsing when broken, but the arteries will constrict to reduce the size of the opening and thereby diminish the loss of blood. Many parts of the body are served by more than one artery, a system called *collateral circulation*. Thus if a blood vessel serving such an area is damaged or restricted, the flow of blood will not stop completely.

1. HEART _____ Purple
2. a. ARCH OF AORTA, b. THORACIC AORTA, and
   c. ABDOMINAL AORTA _____ Pink
3. COMMON ILIAC _____ Orange
4. a. FEMORAL and b. TIBIAL _____ Light Brown
5. SUBCLAVIAN _____ Yellow
6. AXILLARY AND BRACHIAL _____ Green
7. a. ULNAR and b. RADIAL _____ Light Green
8. CAROTID _____ Light Orange
9. VERTEBRAL _____ Brown
10. ARTERIAL BLOOD _____ Red
11. CONNECTIVE TISSUE _____ Light Purple
12. SMOOTH MUSCLE TISSUE _____ Turquoise
13. SEROUS MEMBRANE _____ Flesh

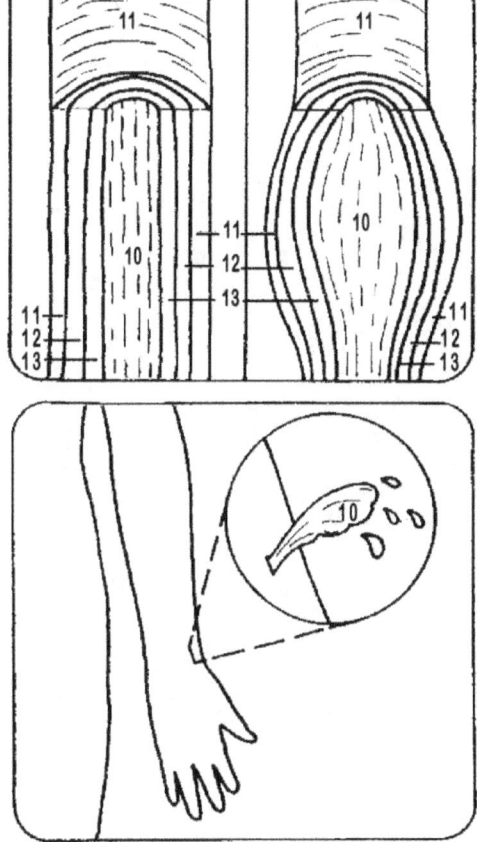

Circulatory System

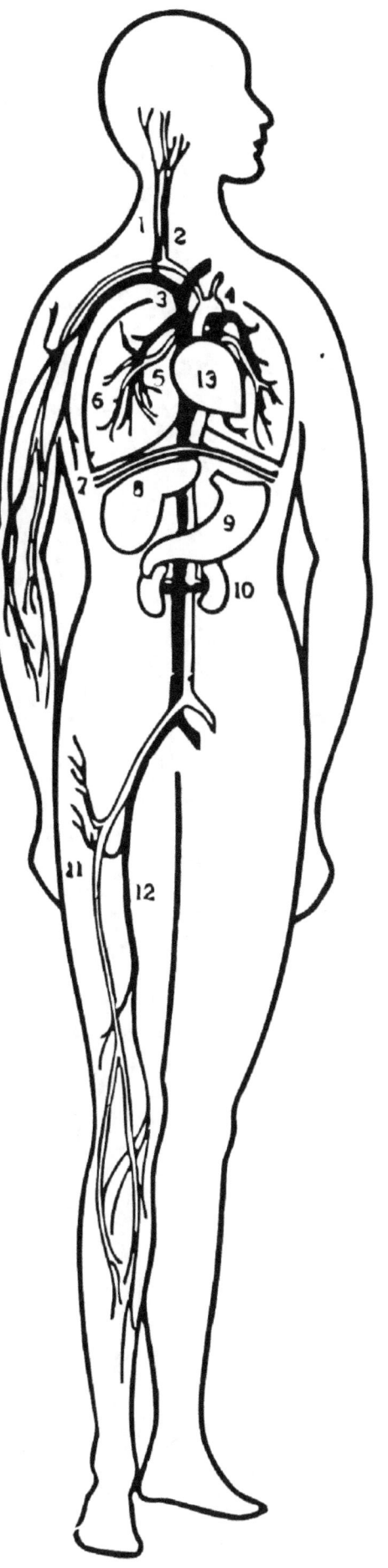

THE CIRCULATORY SYSTEM, ALSO CALLED THE CARDIOVASCULAR SYSTEM OR THE VASCULAR SYSTEM, IS AN ORGAN SYSTEM THAT PERMITS BLOOD TO CIRCULATE AND TRANSPORT NUTRIENTS (SUCH AS AMINO ACIDS AND ELECTROLYTES), OXYGEN, CARBON DIOXIDE, HORMONES, AND BLOOD CELLS TO AND FROM THE CELLS IN THE BODY TO PROVIDE NOURISHMENT AND HELP IN FIGHTING DISEASES, STABILIZE TEMPERATURE AND PH, AND MAINTAIN HOMEOSTASIS.

THE CIRCULATORY SYSTEM INCLUDES THE LYMPHATIC SYSTEM, WHICH CIRCULATES LYMPH. THE PASSAGE OF LYMPH TAKES MUCH LONGER THAN THAT OF BLOOD. BLOOD IS A FLUID CONSISTING OF PLASMA, RED BLOOD CELLS, WHITE BLOOD CELLS, AND PLATELETS THAT IS CIRCULATED BY THE HEART THROUGH THE VERTEBRATE VASCULAR SYSTEM, CARRYING OXYGEN AND NUTRIENTS TO AND WASTE MATERIALS AWAY FROM ALL BODY TISSUES. LYMPH IS ESSENTIALLY RECYCLED EXCESS BLOOD PLASMA AFTER IT HAS BEEN FILTERED FROM THE INTERSTITIAL FLUID (BETWEEN CELLS) AND RETURNED TO THE LYMPHATIC SYSTEM. THE CARDIOVASCULAR (FROM LATIN WORDS MEANING "HEART" AND "VESSEL") SYSTEM COMPRISES THE BLOOD, HEART, AND BLOOD VESSELS.[3] THE LYMPH, LYMPH NODES, AND LYMPH VESSELS FORM THE LYMPHATIC SYSTEM, WHICH RETURNS FILTERED BLOOD PLASMA FROM THE INTERSTITIAL FLUID (BETWEEN CELLS) AS LYMPH.

THE CIRCULATORY SYSTEM OF THE BLOOD IS SEEN AS HAVING TWO COMPONENTS, A SYSTEMIC CIRCULATION AND A PULMONARY CIRCULATION.

WHILE HUMANS, AS WELL AS OTHER VERTEBRATES, HAVE A CLOSED CARDIOVASCULAR SYSTEM (MEANING THAT THE BLOOD NEVER LEAVES THE NETWORK OF ARTERIES, VEINS AND CAPILLARIES), SOME INVERTEBRATE GROUPS HAVE AN OPEN CARDIOVASCULAR SYSTEM. THE LYMPHATIC SYSTEM, ON THE OTHER HAND, IS AN OPEN SYSTEM PROVIDING AN ACCESSORY ROUTE FOR EXCESS INTERSTITIAL FLUID TO BE RETURNED TO THE BLOOD. THE MORE PRIMITIVE, DIPLOBLASTIC ANIMAL PHYLA LACK CIRCULATORY SYSTEMS.

MANY DISEASES AFFECT THE CIRCULATORY SYSTEM. THIS INCLUDES CARDIOVASCULAR DISEASE, AFFECTING THE CARDIOVASCULAR SYSTEM, AND LYMPHATIC DISEASE AFFECTING THE LYMPHATIC SYSTEM. CARDIOLOGISTS ARE MEDICAL PROFESSIONALS WHICH SPECIALISE IN THE HEART, AND CARDIOTHORACIC SURGEONS SPECIALISE IN OPERATING ON THE HEART AND ITS SURROUNDING AREAS. VASCULAR SURGEONS FOCUS ON OTHER PARTS OF THE CIRCULATORY SYSTEM.

1- JUGULAR VEIN —————————————— GREEN
2- CAROTID ARTERIES ————————————— YELLOW
3- SUPERIOR VENA CAVA ——————————— LIGHT PURPLE
4- AORTA ——————————————————— PURPLE
5- PULMONARY ARTERIES ————————————— LIGHT BLUE
6- LUNGS ——————————————————— BROWN
7- DIAPHRAGM ———————————————— PINK
8- LIVER ——————————————————— DARK GREEN
9- STOMACH ————————————————— ORANGE
10- KIDNEYS —————————————————— GREEN
11- FEMORAL ARTERY —————————————— DARK BLUE
12- FEMORAL VEIN ———————————————— TURQUOISE
13- HEART —————————————————— RED

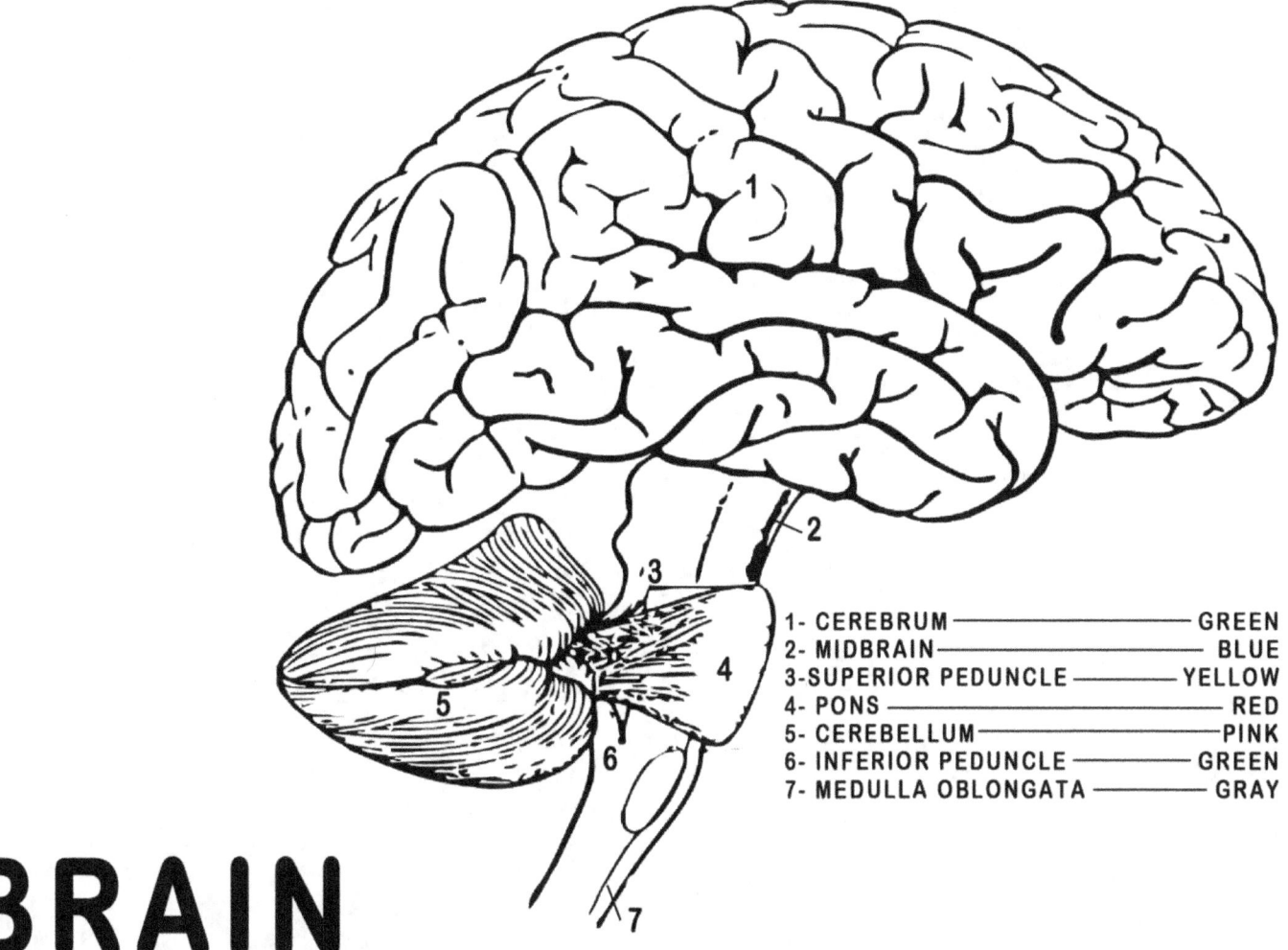

1- CEREBRUM —————— GREEN
2- MIDBRAIN —————— BLUE
3- SUPERIOR PEDUNCLE —— YELLOW
4- PONS —————————— RED
5- CEREBELLUM ————— PINK
6- INFERIOR PEDUNCLE —— GREEN
7- MEDULLA OBLONGATA —— GRAY

BRAIN

THE BRAIN IS AN AMAZING THREE-POUND ORGAN THAT CONTROLS ALL FUNCTIONS OF THE BODY, INTERPRETS INFORMATION FROM THE OUTSIDE WORLD, AND EMBODIES THE ESSENCE OF THE MIND AND SOUL. INTELLIGENCE, CREATIVITY, EMOTION, AND MEMORY ARE A FEW OF THE MANY THINGS GOVERNED BY THE BRAIN. PROTECTED WITHIN THE SKULL, THE BRAIN IS COMPOSED OF THE CEREBRUM, CEREBELLUM, AND BRAINSTEM.

THE BRAIN RECEIVES INFORMATION THROUGH OUR FIVE SENSES: SIGHT, SMELL, TOUCH, TASTE, AND HEARING - OFTEN MANY AT ONE TIME. IT ASSEMBLES THE MESSAGES IN A WAY THAT HAS MEANING FOR US, AND CAN STORE THAT INFORMATION IN OUR MEMORY. THE BRAIN CONTROLS OUR THOUGHTS, MEMORY AND SPEECH, MOVEMENT OF THE ARMS AND LEGS, AND THE FUNCTION OF MANY ORGANS WITHIN OUR BODY.

THE CENTRAL NERVOUS SYSTEM (CNS) IS COMPOSED OF THE BRAIN AND SPINAL CORD. THE PERIPHERAL NERVOUS SYSTEM (PNS) IS COMPOSED OF SPINAL NERVES THAT BRANCH FROM THE SPINAL CORD AND CRANIAL NERVES THAT BRANCH FROM THE BRAIN.

CEREBRUM: IS THE LARGEST PART OF THE BRAIN AND IS COMPOSED OF RIGHT AND LEFT HEMISPHERES. IT PERFORMS HIGHER FUNCTIONS LIKE INTERPRETING TOUCH, VISION AND HEARING, AS WELL AS SPEECH, REASONING, EMOTIONS, LEARNING, AND FINE CONTROL OF MOVEMENT.

CEREBELLUM: IS LOCATED UNDER THE CEREBRUM. ITS FUNCTION IS TO COORDINATE MUSCLE MOVEMENTS, MAINTAIN POSTURE, AND BALANCE.

BRAINSTEM: ACTS AS A RELAY CENTER CONNECTING THE CEREBRUM AND CEREBELLUM TO THE SPINAL CORD. IT PERFORMS MANY AUTOMATIC FUNCTIONS SUCH AS BREATHING, HEART RATE, BODY TEMPERATURE, WAKE AND SLEEP CYCLES, DIGESTION, SNEEZING, COUGHING, VOMITING, AND SWALLOWING.

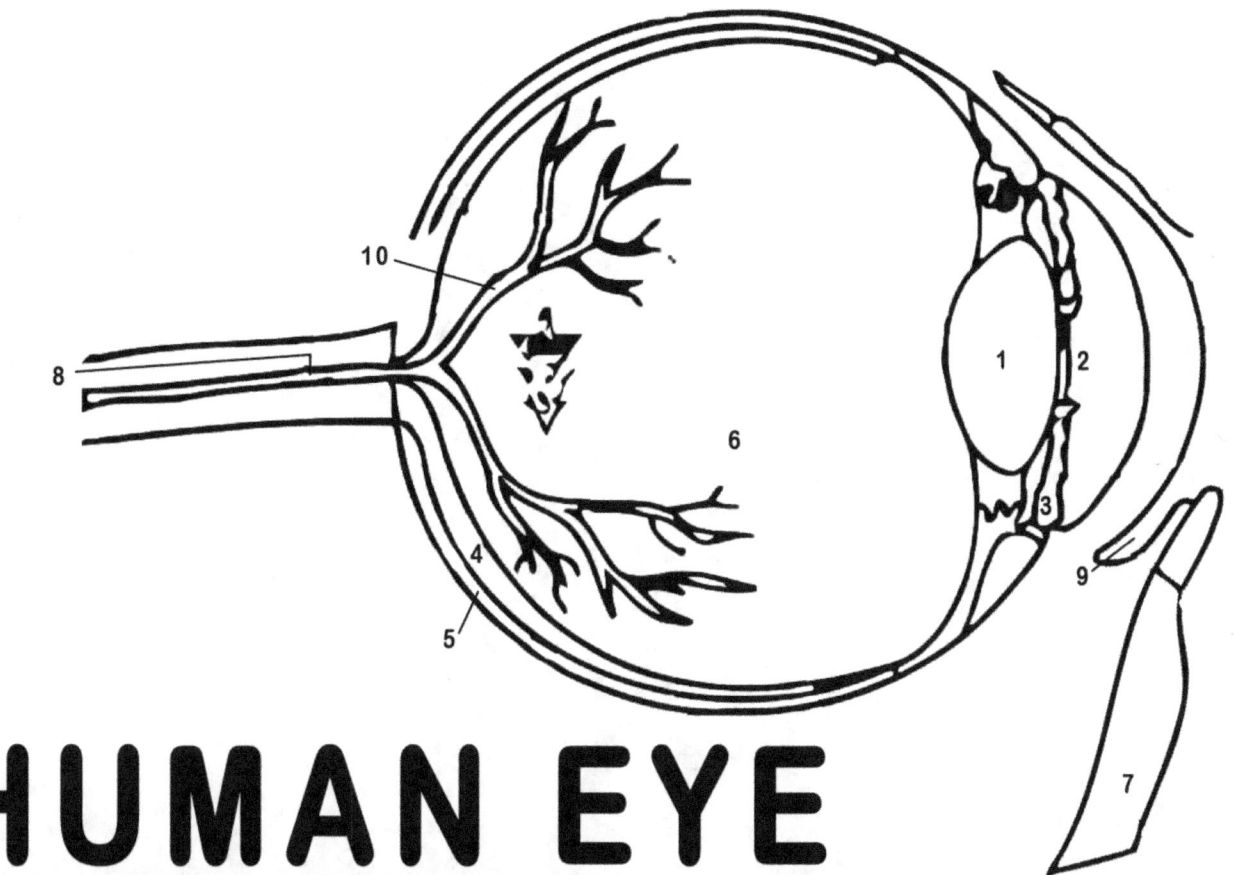

HUMAN EYE

THE HUMAN EYE IS AN ORGAN THAT REACTS TO LIGHT AND ALLOWS VISION. ROD AND CONE CELLS IN THE RETINA ALLOW CONSCIOUS LIGHT PERCEPTION AND VISION INCLUDING COLOR DIFFERENTIATION AND THE PERCEPTION OF DEPTH. THE HUMAN EYE CAN DIFFERENTIATE BETWEEN ABOUT 10 MILLION COLORS AND IS POSSIBLY CAPABLE OF DETECTING A SINGLE PHOTON. THE EYE IS PART OF THE SENSORY NERVOUS SYSTEM.

SIMILAR TO THE EYES OF OTHER MAMMALS, THE HUMAN EYE'S NON-IMAGE-FORMING PHOTOSENSITIVE GANGLION CELLS IN THE RETINA RECEIVE LIGHT SIGNALS WHICH AFFECT ADJUSTMENT OF THE SIZE OF THE PUPIL, REGULATION AND SUPPRESSION OF THE HORMONE MELATONIN AND ENTRAINMENT OF THE BODY

1- LENS —————————————— LIGHT BLUE
2- PUPIL —————————————— GREEN
3- EYELID —————————————— ORANGE
4- RETINA —————————————— PINK
5- CHOROID —————————————— RED
6- VITREOUS HUMOR —————————————— GRAY
7- IRIS —————————————— DARK GREEN
8- OPTIC NERVE —————————————— YELLOW
9- TEAR DUCT —————————————— LIGHT BLUE
10- RETINAL BLOOD VESSELS —————————————— PURPLE

THERE ARE TWO EYES, SITUATED ON THE LEFT AND THE RIGHT OF THE FACE. THEY SIT IN TWO BONY CAVITIES CALLED THE ORBITS, WHICH ARE PRESENT IN THE SKULL. SIX EXTRAOCULAR MUSCLES ATTACH DIRECTLY TO THE EYES TO ASSIST WITH MOVEMENT. THE FRONT VISIBLE PART OF THE EYE IS MADE UP OF THE WHITISH SCLERA, A COLOURED IRIS, AND THE PUPIL. A THIN LAYER CALLED THE CONJUNCTIVA SITS ON TOP OF THIS. THE FRONT PART IS ALSO CALLED THE ANTERIOR SEGMENT OF THE EYE.

THE EYE IS NOT SHAPED LIKE A PERFECT SPHERE, RATHER IT IS A FUSED TWO-PIECE UNIT, COMPOSED OF A ANTERIOR (FRONT) SEGMENT AND THE POSTERIOR (BACK) SEGMENT. THE ANTERIOR SEGMENT IS MADE UP OF THE CORNEA, IRIS AND LENS. THE CORNEA IS TRANSPARENT AND MORE CURVED, AND IS LINKED TO THE LARGER POSTERIOR SEGMENT, COMPOSED OF THE VITREOUS, RETINA, CHOROID AND THE OUTER WHITE SHELL CALLED THE SCLERA. THE CORNEA IS TYPICALLY ABOUT 11.5 MM (0.3 IN) IN DIAMETER, AND 0.5 MM (500 μM) IN THICKNESS NEAR ITS CENTER. THE POSTERIOR CHAMBER CONSTITUTES THE REMAINING FIVE-SIXTHS; ITS DIAMETER IS TYPICALLY ABOUT 24 MM. THE CORNEA AND SCLERA ARE CONNECTED BY AN AREA TERMED THE LIMBUS. THE IRIS IS THE PIGMENTED CIRCULAR STRUCTURE CONCENTRICALLY SURROUNDING THE CENTER OF THE EYE, THE PUPIL, WHICH APPEARS TO BE BLACK. THE SIZE OF THE PUPIL, WHICH CONTROLS THE AMOUNT OF LIGHT ENTERING THE EYE, IS ADJUSTED BY THE IRIS' DILATOR AND SPHINCTER MUSCLES.

Anatomy of the Artery

CHOOSE YOUR OWN COLORS

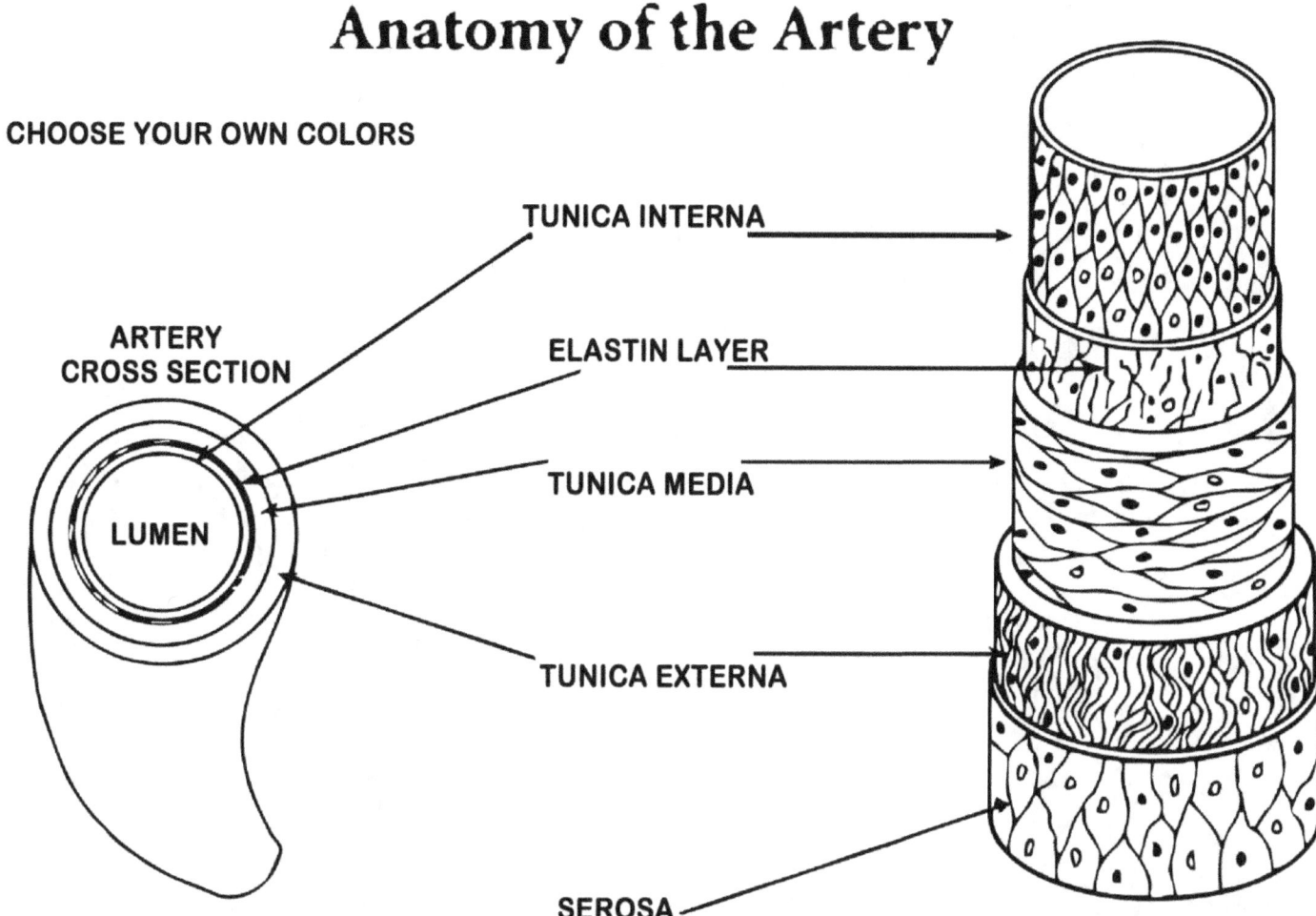

Labels: ARTERY CROSS SECTION, LUMEN, TUNICA INTERNA, ELASTIN LAYER, TUNICA MEDIA, TUNICA EXTERNA, SEROSA

THE ARTERIES ARE THE BLOOD VESSELS THAT DELIVER OXYGEN-RICH BLOOD FROM THE HEART TO THE TISSUES OF THE BODY. EACH ARTERY IS A MUSCULAR TUBE LINED BY SMOOTH TISSUE AND HAS THREE LAYERS:

-THE INTIMA, THE INNER LAYER LINED BY A SMOOTH TISSUE CALLED ENDOTHELIUM

-THE MEDIA, A LAYER OF MUSCLE THAT LETS ARTERIES HANDLE THE HIGH PRESSURES FROM THE HEART

-THE ADVENTITIA, CONNECTIVE TISSUE ANCHORING ARTERIES TO NEARBY TISSUES

THE LARGEST ARTERY IS THE AORTA, THE MAIN HIGH-PRESSURE PIPELINE CONNECTED TO THE HEART'S LEFT VENTRICLE. THE AORTA BRANCHES INTO A NETWORK OF SMALLER ARTERIES THAT EXTEND THROUGHOUT THE BODY. THE ARTERIES' SMALLER BRANCHES ARE CALLED ARTERIOLES AND CAPILLARIES. THE PULMONARY ARTERIES CARRY OXYGEN-POOR BLOOD FROM THE HEART TO THE LUNGS UNDER LOW PRESSURE, MAKING THESE ARTERIES UNIQUE.

CONDITIONS OF THE ARTERIES

ATHEROSCLEROSIS: THE BUILDUP OF CHOLESTEROL (A WAXY SUBSTANCE) INTO WHAT ARE CALLED PLAQUES IN THE ARTERIES' WALLS. ATHEROSCLEROSIS IN THE ARTERIES OF THE HEART, BRAIN, OR NECK CAN LEAD TO HEART ATTACKS AND STROKES.

VASCULITIS (ARTERITIS): INFLAMMATION OF THE ARTERIES, WHICH MAY INVOLVE ONE OR MORE ARTERIES AT THE SAME TIME. MOST VASCULITIS IS CAUSED BY AN OVERACTIVE IMMUNE SYSTEM.

AMAUROSIS FUGAX: LOSS OF VISION IN ONE EYE CAUSED BY A TEMPORARY LOSS OF BLOOD FLOW TO THE RETINA, THE LIGHT-SENSITIVE TISSUE THAT LINES THE BACK OF THE EYE. IT USUALLY OCCURS WHEN A PORTION OF A CHOLESTEROL PLAQUE IN ONE OF THE CAROTID ARTERIES (THE ARTERIES ON EITHER SIDE OF THE NECK THAT SUPPLY BLOOD TO THE BRAIN) BREAKS OFF AND TRAVELS TO THE RETINAL ARTERY (THE ARTERY THAT SUPPLIES BLOOD AND NUTRIENTS TO THE RETINA.)

TOOTH ANATOMY

TEETH CONDITIONS

THE TEETH ARE THE HARDEST SUBSTANCES IN THE HUMAN BODY. BESIDES BEING ESSENTIAL FOR CHEWING, THE TEETH PLAY AN IMPORTANT ROLE IN SPEECH. PARTS OF THE TEETH INCLUDE:

ENAMEL: THE HARDEST, WHITE OUTER PART OF THE TOOTH. ENAMEL IS MOSTLY MADE OF CALCIUM PHOSPHATE, A ROCK-HARD MINERAL.

DENTIN: A LAYER UNDERLYING THE ENAMEL. IT IS A HARD TISSUE THAT CONTAINS MICROSCOPIC TUBES. WHEN THE ENAMEL IS DAMAGED, HEAT OR COLD CAN ENTER THE TOOTH THROUGH THESE PATHS AND CAUSE SENSITIVITY OR PAIN.

PULP: THE SOFTER, LIVING INNER STRUCTURE OF TEETH. BLOOD VESSELS AND NERVES RUN THROUGH THE PULP OF THE TEETH.

CEMENTUM: A LAYER OF CONNECTIVE TISSUE THAT BINDS THE ROOTS OF THE TEETH FIRMLY TO THE GUMS AND JAWBONE.

PERIODONTAL LIGAMENT: TISSUE THAT HELPS HOLD THE TEETH TIGHTLY AGAINST THE JAW.

A NORMAL ADULT MOUTH HAS 32 TEETH, WHICH (EXCEPT FOR WISDOM TEETH) HAVE ERUPTED BY ABOUT AGE 13:

• INCISORS (8 TOTAL): THE MIDDLEMOST FOUR TEETH ON THE UPPER AND LOWER JAWS.
• CANINES (4 TOTAL): THE POINTED TEETH JUST OUTSIDE THE INCISORS.
• PREMOLARS (8 TOTAL): TEETH BETWEEN THE CANINES AND MOLARS.
• MOLARS (8 TOTAL): FLAT TEETH IN THE REAR OF THE MOUTH, BEST AT GRINDING FOOD.
• WISDOM TEETH OR THIRD MOLARS (4 TOTAL): THESE TEETH ERUPT AT AROUND AGE 18, BUT ARE OFTEN SURGICALLY REMOVED TO PREVENT DISPLACEMENT OF OTHER TEETH.

CAVITIES (CARIES): BACTERIA EVADE REMOVAL BY BRUSHING AND SALIVA AND DAMAGE THE ENAMEL AND DEEPER STRUCTURES OF TEETH. MOST CAVITIES OCCUR ON MOLARS AND PREMOLARS.

TOOTH DECAY: A GENERAL NAME FOR DISEASE OF THE TEETH, INCLUDING CAVITIES.

PERIODONTITIS: INFLAMMATION OF THE DEEPER STRUCTURES OF THE TEETH (PERIODONTAL LIGAMENT, JAWBONE, AND CEMENTUM). POOR ORAL HYGIENE IS USUALLY TO BLAME.

GINGIVITIS: INFLAMMATION OF THE SURFACE PORTION OF THE GUMS, AROUND AND BETWEEN THE CROWNS OF THE TEETH. PLAQUE AND TARTAR BUILDUP CAN LEAD TO GINGIVITIS.

PLAQUE: A STICKY, COLORLESS FILM MADE OF BACTERIA AND THE SUBSTANCES THEY SECRETE. PLAQUE DEVELOPS QUICKLY ON TEETH AFTER EATING SUGARY FOOD, BUT CAN BE EASILY BRUSHED OFF.

TARTAR: IF PLAQUE IS NOT REMOVED, IT MIXES WITH MINERALS TO BECOME TARTAR, A HARDER SUBSTANCE. TARTAR REQUIRES PROFESSIONAL CLEANING FOR REMOVAL.

OVERBITE: THE UPPER TEETH PROTRUDE SIGNIFICANTLY OVER THE LOWER TEETH.

UNDERBITE: THE LOWER TEETH PROTRUDE SIGNIFICANTLY PAST THE UPPER TEETH.

TEETH GRINDING (BRUXISM): STRESS, ANXIETY, OR SLEEP DISORDERS CAN CAUSE TEETH GRINDING, USUALLY DURING SLEEP. A DULL HEADACHE OR SORE JAW CAN BE SYMPTOMS.

TOOTH SENSITIVITY: WHEN ONE OR MORE TEETH BECOME SENSITIVE TO HOT OR COLD, IT MAY MEAN THE DENTIN IS EXPOSED.

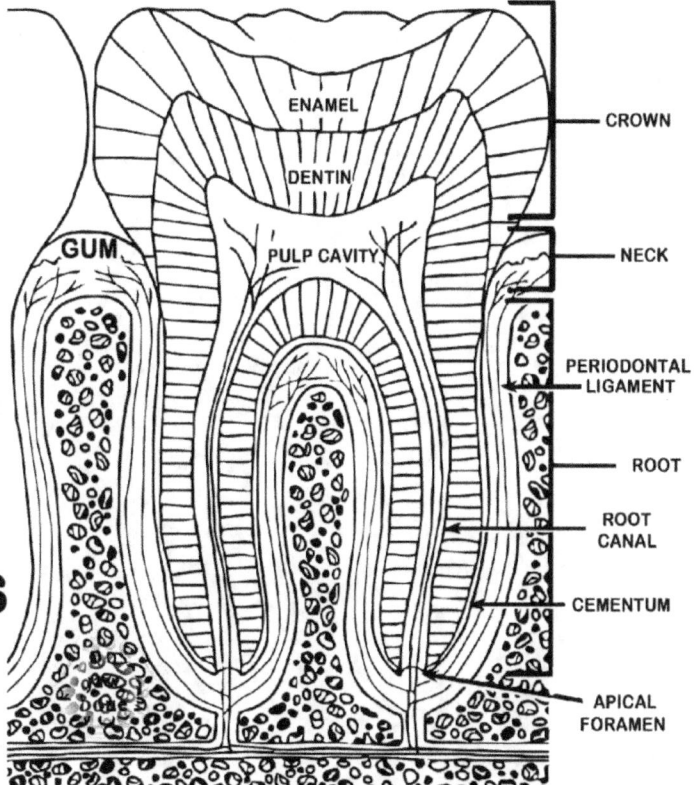

CHOOSE YOUR OWN COLORS

Integumentary System: *skin, hair, nails, and glands*

1 - epidermis
2 - dermis
3 - hypodermis
4 - hair follicle
5 - sebaceous (oil) gland
6 - blood vessels
7 - sweat gland
8 - touch receptors
9 - pore

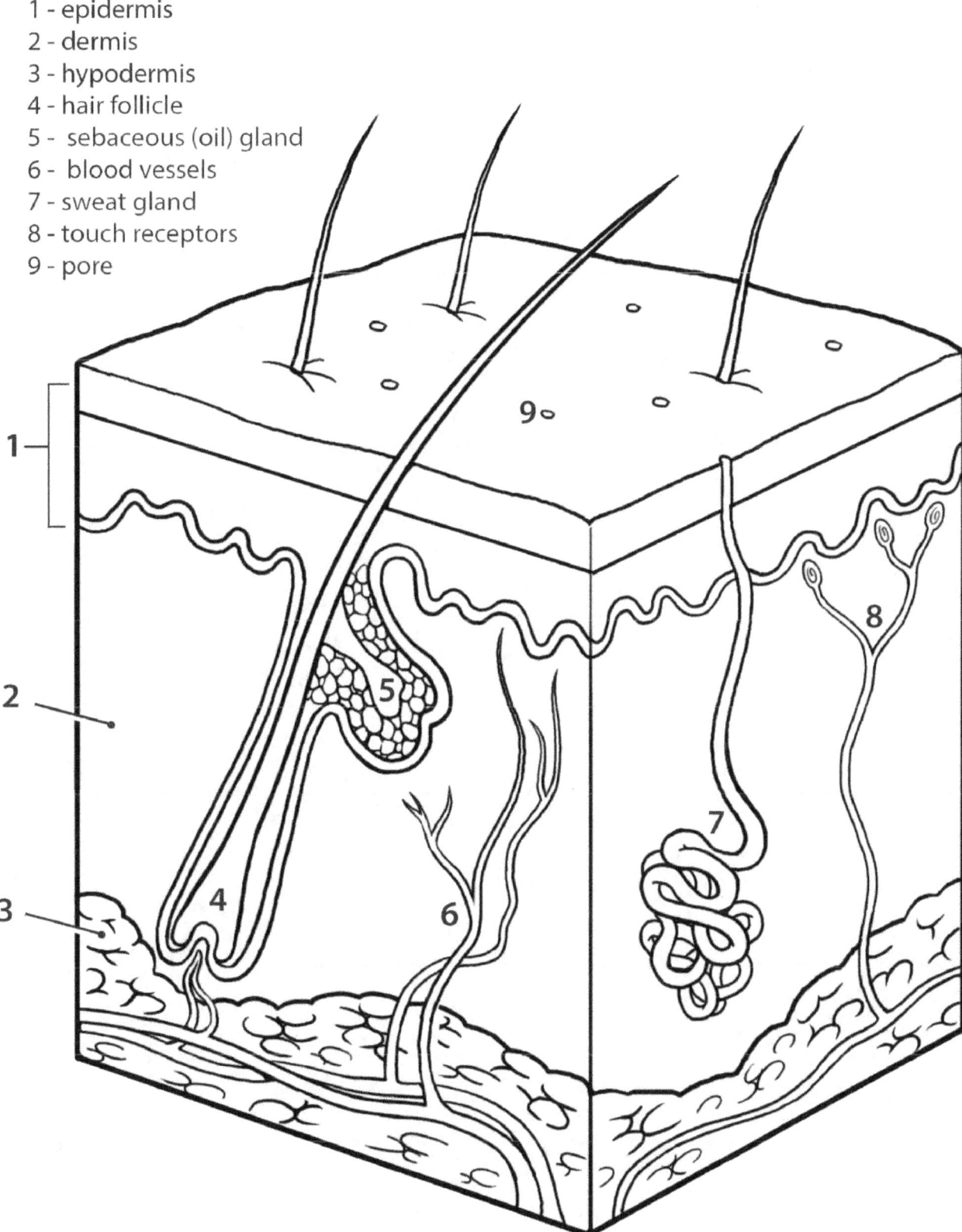

Parts of the Ear

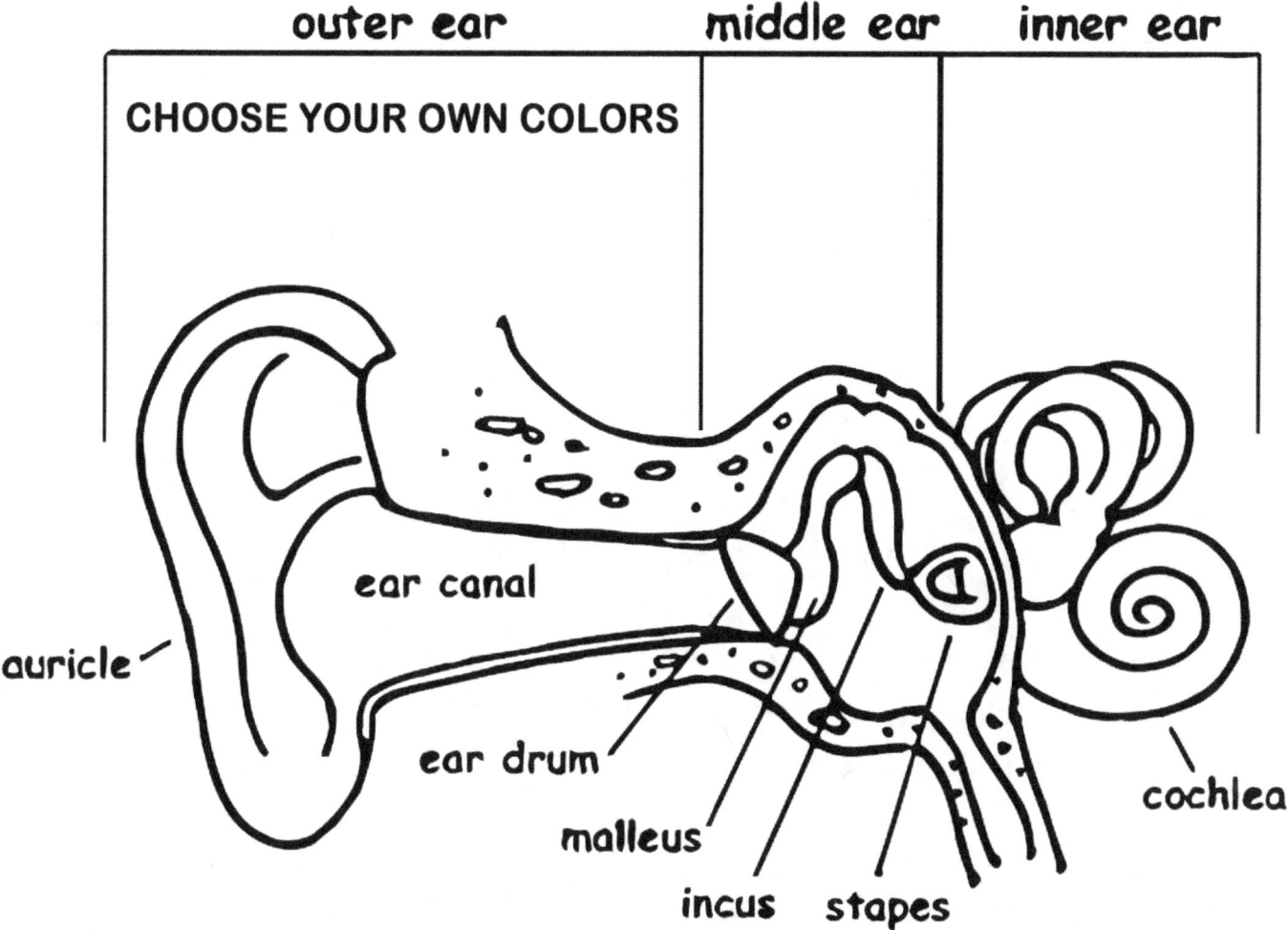

THE EAR IS THE ORGAN OF HEARING AND, IN MAMMALS, BALANCE. IN MAMMALS, THE EAR IS USUALLY DESCRIBED AS HAVING THREE PARTS—THE OUTER EAR, THE MIDDLE EAR AND THE INNER EAR. THE OUTER EAR CONSISTS OF THE PINNA AND THE EAR CANAL. SINCE THE OUTER EAR IS THE ONLY VISIBLE PORTION OF THE EAR IN MOST ANIMALS, THE WORD "EAR" OFTEN REFERS TO THE EXTERNAL PART ALONE. THE MIDDLE EAR INCLUDES THE TYMPANIC CAVITY AND THE THREE OSSICLES. THE INNER EAR SITS IN THE BONY LABYRINTH, AND CONTAINS STRUCTURES WHICH ARE KEY TO SEVERAL SENSES: THE SEMICIRCULAR CANALS, WHICH ENABLE BALANCE AND EYE TRACKING WHEN MOVING; THE UTRICLE AND SACCULE, WHICH ENABLE BALANCE WHEN STATIONARY; AND THE COCHLEA, WHICH ENABLES HEARING. THE EARS OF VERTEBRATES ARE PLACED SOMEWHAT SYMMETRICALLY ON EITHER SIDE OF THE HEAD, AN ARRANGEMENT THAT AIDS SOUND LOCALISATION.

THE EAR DEVELOPS FROM THE FIRST PHARYNGEAL POUCH AND SIX SMALL SWELLINGS THAT DEVELOP IN THE EARLY EMBRYO CALLED OTIC PLACODES, WHICH ARE DERIVED FROM ECTODERM.

THE EAR MAY BE AFFECTED BY DISEASE, INCLUDING INFECTION AND TRAUMATIC DAMAGE. DISEASES OF THE EAR MAY LEAD TO HEARING LOSS, TINNITUS AND BALANCE DISORDERS SUCH AS VERTIGO, ALTHOUGH MANY OF THESE CONDITIONS MAY ALSO BE AFFECTED BY DAMAGE TO THE BRAIN OR NEURAL PATHWAYS LEADING FROM THE EAR.

PLEASE IF YOU LIKE THE BOOK, GIVE ME 5 STARS AND COMMENT FOR SUPPORT

www.ingramcontent.com/pod-product-compliance
Lightning Source LLC
Chambersburg PA
CBHW080953220526
45465CB00008BA/3264